HOW TO
Grow a Baby*

*and Push it Out

For Anya, Marnie, Ottilie and Delilah,
the greatest girl gang a mother could have asked for.

HOW TO

Grow a Baby*

*and Push it Out

Your no-nonsense guide
to pregnancy and birth

Clemmie Hooper

MIDWIFE

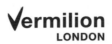

Vermilion
LONDON

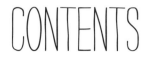

CONTENTS

Introduction

INTRODUCTION

Having been a midwife for over ten years and given birth to four of my own children (sometimes I still can't believe I have four children), I would like to think that I have now gained enough experience and knowledge to write a whole book on being pregnant and giving birth.

In truth, this book won't tell you absolutely everything you need to know because you'd need more than an entire pregnancy to read that. But it will tell you about the important stuff, the stuff which some people skim over, and it will also tell you about things that you may be too embarrassed to ask your midwife (although you should know that you can ask your midwife anything – rest assured, they will have heard it before). This book is written by me, your midwife, and each chapter is based around the key stages and routine antenatal appointments you will be offered. I will address how to cope in those early days before anyone else knows, what to expect when going for your 12-week scan, coping with the emotional changes you may experience during those nine months, and what you really need to pack in your hospital bag for when the big day arrives.

I've helped hundreds of women through their individual journeys into motherhood, whether it's their first time or they've done it several times before. I've seen it all – from home births (planned and unplanned), water births, births in the back of a taxi, inductions and C-sections. I've delivered sets of twins (including my own) and seen triplets being born, and sadly helped deliver babies too premature to survive. Yet each birth, no matter how that baby is born, still fills me with the same feelings of emotion and amazement and what an honour it is, as a midwife, to be part of every single one of those life-changing moments.

I wrote this book so you can feel empowered. By giving you all the information you need to understand what options are available to you, I hope that you can go on to make informed choices about how you will experience the birth of your baby so it's the right birth for you. You don't have to do what your best friend did or listen to that woman from work – your birth experience should be as unique as you are. Remember that women have been giving birth since the beginning of time and so we should learn to trust our bodies and know that birth doesn't have to be scary or stressful. Yes, pregnancy is full of ups and downs and it's unlikely to be perfect and amazing all the way along, but that's just part of the beauty of it – each experience is different and I hope this book can help you ride out any of those lows along with all of the highs.

Throughout the book you'll also come across personal birth stories from real mums, each one totally different but each one full of really useful information you can take away and apply to the preparation for your own birth experience. By the time you finish reading this book I hope you will feel excited and full of confidence that whatever birth you have, it will be the most positive birth for you. Every birth I've attended was as beautiful and special as the others, and I want to share what I have learnt in this book to help you realise that your own birth story will be just as amazing.

Clemmie
x

10 WEEKS

IN THE BEGINNING

YOUR BABY IS ABOUT THE SIZE OF A STRAWBERRY.
IT IS A LITTLE OVER 3CM LONG AND WEIGHS ABOUT 4G.

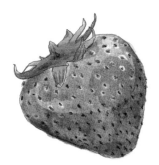

THE TWO PINK LINES

You've made it! Congratulations! How you got here is different from woman to woman; it may have been a one-night stand, years of infertility, a sperm donor from a clinic or the bog-standard way of just having unprotected sex with your partner. But whatever your story, you're here now and you've probably got a million thoughts and questions racing through your mind.

SLOW DOWN. It's only the beginning. You need this whole pregnancy to get your head around the fact that you're going to be a mother. There will be a baby (or babies) at the end of this journey, so take your time, ask questions and surround yourself in positivity. Everyone will give you their tips, advice and opinions: just take it all with a pinch of salt. Only you know your own mind. Even if your emotions are all over the place (hormones are a funny thing!), take a breather and focus on one thing at a time. Even if that's what to make for dinner! There's plenty of time to think about the bigger picture.

Don't panic about things like 'what sort of birth do I want?'. You can address these mind-boggling questions when you have more information as your pregnancy develops and you start finding out more about your options. I often tell women you can't 'plan' your birth anyway, so let go of the things you can't control and just get through these next few weeks. Rest and nurture your changing body: it's doing an incredible thing growing a tiny human.

When I found out I was unexpectedly pregnant with my first baby at 23, I stared at the pregnancy test for what felt like an hour. I kept turning it over and looking at it, hoping it had miraculously changed from positive to negative. But, of course, it hadn't: it was a big fat positive. Those two pink lines staring at me on that plastic stick suddenly meant my plans would change for ever. So don't worry if you too are feeling overwhelmed by what lies ahead. It's entirely normal, even if this pregnancy was planned. Hopefully this book will support and guide you through it all. Think of it as your go-to for all those niggling questions you may be too afraid to even ask your mum.

One of the most frequent questions I get asked as a midwife is: 'I've been on a bender and didn't realise I was pregnant! Will my baby be okay?'

Fear not, ladies, you are not alone if you find yourself in this situation. There's obviously not a huge amount you can do at this stage, but feeling guilty and worrying about it isn't going to change anything either. Feel reassured that lots of mums start off their pregnancy in exactly the same way:

> I had my 30th birthday the weekend before I found out I was pregnant! I was so scared that there would be some lasting effects of the alcohol I drank on my unborn baby. While pregnant I reassured myself by thinking about how I'm sure I wasn't alone in my circumstances and that managed to tame the guilt I was feeling.
>
> *Sophie, mum of two*

But as soon as you find out you are pregnant, stop drinking any alcohol. The Chief Medical Officers for the UK (NHS.uk) recommend that if you're pregnant, or planning to become pregnant, to keep risks to your baby to a minimum the safest approach is not to drink alcohol at all.

Try to let go of the guilt and things you can't change and focus on the things you can do from now on: eating well, taking the right supplements and resting. I found pregnancy to be the best and biggest detox I've ever been on!

Think about ways to live more healthily. If you're used to exercising, whether that's swimming, running or cycling to work, and still feel like doing it, then go for it! There is no evidence that suggests that continuing your normal exercise routine is more likely to cause harm to you or your baby. I wouldn't recommend suddenly taking up a new high-impact sport as your body won't be used to it, so stick to what you're used to, especially if it makes you feel good! Endorphins are good for you, after all.

Most importantly, relax and try to enjoy the next few months. This first chapter will take you through those early stages so you can feel more prepared for the next part of your pregnancy.

THINGS YOU SHOULD BE DOING NOW

I've compiled a list of things you should be doing by now, but don't worry if you haven't done them all yet. Tick the things you can achieve and make a note of the things you will try to do by, say, week 10. Remember, it's early days and there is plenty of time.

- If you haven't already, pee on a stick to confirm you're actually pregnant. If you're very unsure of the first day of your last period you may need to have an early dating scan, which your GP can arrange for you.
- Make a doctor's appointment. This should be the first health professional you see. He or she will arrange your 12-week scan and your first midwife appointment.
- Once you've worked out your estimated due date, I recommend only telling people on a need-to-know basis (see page 15). And by that I mean your midwife and partner. I would also strongly recommend you add a week on to your pregnancy when telling friends and family. Only 5 per cent of babies are born on their due date. Your cycle may not even be exactly 28 days so you may not ovulate on day 14. Surprisingly, you are not a bag of microwave popcorn that will pop at 40 weeks.
- Start taking folic acid (400mcg per day) if you haven't already. Folic acid helps to protect your unborn baby from neural tubal defects such as spina bifida. Once you are 13 weeks' pregnant there is no need to continue taking the supplement.
- If you're suffering from morning sickness (see pages 18–19) and are finding it hard to get all the right goodness into your diet because you're surviving on cheese on toast, you may want to think about taking some multivitamins. Check the list of ingredients carefully, as some vitamins, such as Vitamin A, aren't recommended in pregnancy.
- You may also want to take extra iron at this point. That tiny fetus and developing placenta have a very clever way of stealing all your iron stores

12

from you, and if you're still finding it hard to keep anything down, an extra iron tablet a day could make all the difference to your energy levels.

- Early pregnancy can be hard, both physically and emotionally. Motivating yourself to do any exercise can be challenging, especially when all you want to do is curl up and eat crisps. But exercise can be anything from swimming and cycling to pregnancy yoga, gentle running or even just a good walk. So get moving. (See pages 11 and 49 for more on this.)

- Avoid that litter tray. If you have a cat that uses a litter tray the good news is you can – and should – pass over that job to your partner. Cat poo can contain a parasite called toxoplasmosis. Although very rare, it can cause a miscarriage. If you do any gardening, remember to wear gloves in case you come into contact with cat poo and always wash your hands thoroughly.

- Fill out an FW8 form, which your GP or midwife will give you. This entitles you to free prescriptions until your baby's first birthday. You will then be sent a card that you show to the pharmacy every time you collect a prescription.

- Find an NHS dentist. More good news – you also get free dental care and treatments up until your baby turns one. This is especially important as you're more likely to suffer from bleeding and swollen gums in pregnancy. So there's no better time to get that toothache looked at!

- If you are working, find out what Maternity Pay you're entitled to. Legally you don't have to tell work you're pregnant yet (and you may want to wait until after your 12-week scan) but planning your finances in advance is a really good idea. Check out www.gov.uk/pay-leave-for-parents to calculate what you're entitled to.

- And last, but not least: go easy on yourself. Your body is doing a huge amount of work, even in these early weeks, so don't be surprised at how exhausted you may be feeling. Getting home from work and having a kip on the sofa is absolutely fine: your body obviously needs it. And if, like me, you have young children to tend to while attempting to make a nutritious evening meal (fish fingers are totally acceptable, by the way) see if your partner can get home a bit earlier than usual to share the load. Remember that this phase of exhaustion won't last for ever and never underestimate how incredible you are!

WHAT ANTENATAL CARE?

Confused? It's not surprising that women are often left feeling overwhelmed by all the information thrown at them. I've simplified the four different types of antenatal care you can expect to receive here in the UK to help you navigate your way towards choosing what's right for you and your baby.

- **Midwifery care**: For women who are low-risk (see page 62 for more on what this means). You are looked after by your own midwife or team of midwives. This is sometimes called 'one-to-one' care or team 'midwifery' care. It's not offered in all parts of the country, so speak to your GP about your options. Midwives see you for all your routine antenatal appointments and care for you during your labour and postnatally. You still have standard scans carried out by sonographers at the hospital.
- **Shared care**: This is the most common. Women are cared for by their GP and community midwife during pregnancy, with visits to the hospital limited to scans or investigating problems. Care is transferred to the hospital for the birth (including home birth), and back to the doctor/midwife afterwards.
- **Consultant care:** Women with pre-existing medical problems and women who are over forty may have regular checks with a hospital-based consultant and all their care may need to be carried out in hospital. There are some conditions, such as diabetes, that require the care of two specialists: an expert in the medical condition as well as an obstetrician.
- **Independent midwives**: Some women prefer to be cared for by an independent midwife who charges a fee for care during pregnancy, at the birth and afterwards. See: www.independentmidwives.org.uk

The exact number of antenatal appointments you have and how often you have them will depend on your situation. If you are expecting your first child, you are likely to have up to ten appointments. If you have had children before, you should have around seven appointments.

So, as soon as you have got over some of the shock that you are pregnant, make an appointment to see your GP, who can discuss what antenatal care is available in your area and set you up with dates for your various next steps. They will also assign you a hospital – usually the one closest to where you live, but the options vary depending on where you're located. Your 'booking' appointment with your midwife will then be arranged – usually by 10 weeks into your pregnancy.

Visit these websites for more information on next steps:

www.nice.org.uk/guidance/cg62/chapter/appendix-d-antenatal-appointments-schedule-and-content

www.nhs.uk/conditions/pregnancy-and-baby/pages/antenatal-midwife-care-pregnant.aspx

TO TELL OR NOT TO TELL

Keeping such an exciting secret can be really difficult. It can feel exhausting constantly deceiving people as to why you're not drinking, staying out late or eating certain foods. Even so, many couples choose not to tell anyone until they've had their 12-week scan and have been reassured that all is well.

But sometimes a problem aired is a problem shared. Some women find that telling closest friends who have had a baby already reassures them that certain things are 'normal'. Some people are also more open to telling close friends/family before the 12-week scan because if anything does go wrong and they miscarry, those are the very people they would call on for support.

Whatever you choose to do, make sure you and your partner are both happy with the decision. Pregnancy can make those closest to you react in all sorts of funny ways, including being miffed at who was told first. And of course there will always be those friends who are struggling to conceive. But try not to let this worry you too much; this is an exciting time for you.

DIET DOS AND DON'TS

Don't panic! Morning sickness permitting (see pages 18–19), you can still eat most of your favourite foods while pregnant, with a couple of tweaks here and there. There's no need to go mad memorising endless lists; just be sensible and realistic.

Bear in mind that we're all different shapes and sizes, and some of us are more active than others. So any recommendation about the quantity of calories you need when you're pregnant is based on averages and your lifestyle. You don't need any more calories than normal until you reach the third trimester; even then you only need 200 extra per day.

- Beware rare: Cook everything thoroughly, including meat, eggs and seafood. Steak and prawns are still on the menu, but only if they're well done. And remember: no runny eggs with your soldiers!
- Check your cheese: Most cheeses are fine in pregnancy. Just avoid soft blue cheeses such as Gorgonzola and mould-ripened cheeses like Camembert, Brie and chèvre (soft goat's cheese). This is because these 'wetter' cheeses are more likely to breed listeria, a type of bacteria that can give you food poisoning. Bake them, though, and problem solved – so pop them on a pizza or bake a Camembert whole.
- Park the pâté: All pâté, even vegetarian pâté, is off the menu as they are also considered a high-listeria risk.
- Curb your caffeine: Drinking two cups of tea OR one cup of coffee a day keeps you under the recommended limit. But watch out for extra shots if you grab your coffee on the go: buy it from a coffee shop or café and you could be drinking more caffeine than you think.
- Think fish: Oily fish such as salmon, fresh tuna and mackerel are good for you, but limit them to twice a week. This is because bigger fish like these eat smaller fish so build up higher levels of mercury. Limit tinned tuna to 4 tins (160g each) per week for the same reason.

- Supermarket-safe zone: Cured meat like Parma ham and chorizo and cured fish such as smoked salmon are fine as long as you buy them from a supermarket. This is because the big stores freeze everything, which kills any possible parasites. Delis and restaurants may not freeze things first, so if in doubt, don't – or ask.
- Leave the liver alone: Admittedly not many people eat liver nowadays but you may eat liver pâté or take cod liver oil, which are also no-nos. Liver is rich in Vitamin A (preformed or retinol), which can cause birth defects, so best leave well alone.
- Say bye bye to alcohol: The chances are you'd probably heave at the thought of drinking a glass of your favourite Soave at the moment, but once the seasick feeling has settled things may change. The recommendation from the RCOG (Royal College of Obstetricians and Gynaecologists) is that during early pregnancy, the safest approach is to abstain from alcohol entirely. After the first trimester, if you do decide to have an alcoholic drink, keep within the recommended amounts: women are advised not to drink more than one to two units more than once or twice a week.
- Don't go nuts about not eating nuts: It's absolutely fine to eat peanuts during pregnancy, unless of course you're allergic to them yourself. There's no evidence that eating peanuts, or foods containing peanuts, while you're pregnant affects, whether or not your baby develops a peanut allergy.

MORNING SICKNESS

Why is it called 'morning sickness' when I feel sick all day? It is estimated that around three-quarters of women experience feeling nauseous in early pregnancy, usually starting at around six weeks. It can strike at any time of day, so the term 'morning' is a bit misleading if, like me, you only feel sick in the evenings. It's probably one of the worst early symptoms of pregnancy as it can really make simple things difficult, such as enjoying meals, travelling to work and sitting through those all-important meetings. It can also make trying to hide your pregnancy from others difficult – depending on their nosiness!

But why do I feel so sick? A little bit of biology here to help you understand why you may be feeling so green around the gills. It is not exactly clear why women experience morning sickness, but it is thought to be connected to the hormones being produced in large quantities in your body. Production of these hormones, HCG (human chorionic gonadotrophin) and oestrogen is then taken over by the placenta once it has grown enough to take over nourishing your baby. So try to remember that it is a good sign and trust your body to do its job caring for your tiny little baby. However, if you're one of those lucky women who don't experience a second of sickness, don't worry that all is not well, because your body will still be doing a great job at making sure everything is developing normally. You're just lucky!

How can I get through the next six weeks? It really is miserable feeling sick and some women may actually vomit too. If you're still in the early stages of pregnancy and for whatever reason don't want to tell friends and family yet, you need to know how to hide the symptoms and deal with them. Lots of women I have looked after in pregnancy all agreed that the best thing to do was eat – they all felt that if their stomach was empty the nausea was worse. So even if you wake up not feeling sick, make sure you eat something straight away. A banana, piece of toast with honey, or a digestive biscuit are all good things that are easy to digest. Lots of women find having snacks in their bag to nibble on if they're commuting is helpful, as feeling like you're going to vomit while stuck on the underground or on the bus is no fun. And always ensure you have a bottle of water handy: small sips are vital to head off dehydration. See over the page for more tips from a health writer who might be able to help you through this tough time.

All I'm eating is beige food. How can I ensure I'm getting the right nutrients to my baby? I remember being told that those first 12 weeks of pregnancy feel like one long hangover; you're tired; you eat the wrong foods and feel a mix of nauseous and bloated. So it can be difficult to eat healthy foods when most of them make you gag. Try to remember that this won't last for ever and in your second trimester (13–28 weeks) you're likely to start eating well again, as you begin to feel much better. If you manage to get one piece of fruit or veg into your daily diet then you are doing better than most. Remember: if you've eaten a good pre-pregnancy diet then you've laid down the important pre-conception nutrients in your system. So try not to worry too much as you'll make up for it later in pregnancy when your body will be saying 'I'm starving' and you can really start to enjoy the taste of flavoured foods again. I couldn't wait to enjoy eating meals with flavours and spice in them, having previously lived on jacket potatoes and chunks of cucumber.

I'm vomiting up to 20 times a day and can hardly keep anything down, including water. Is this normal? This is hyperemesis gravidarum, which means excessive vomiting in pregnancy. The severity of the vomiting can cause dehydration, weight loss and a build-up of toxins in the blood or urine called ketosis. It affects nearly 4 per 1,000 pregnant women and can cause women to vomit blood. If you're experiencing excessive vomiting and are unable to keep even water down, it's best to go straight to your GP, where you will be asked to provide a urine sample and have a blood test to make sure you're not too dehydrated. In some cases it may be recommended that you are admitted to hospital to have IV (intravenous) fluids, such as saline, and kept in for observation. Some women are also prescribed anti-sickness medicine to take until the symptoms have improved. Even though hyperemesis is truly horrible and makes you feel awful, it is very unlikely that any harm will come to your baby.

FIGHT THE URGE TO PURGE

EMMA BARDWELL, HEALTH AND WELLNESS
WRITER, @80PERCENTCLEAN

The term 'morning sickness' is a something of a misnomer. As anyone who has suffered from this debilitating affliction will tell you, it rarely limits itself to the hours before noon. The harsh truth is, it can strike at any time. For most women it starts around week 6 and usually tails off around weeks 12–14 but, for an unfortunate few, it can carry on throughout the pregnancy. Here are a few pointers and easy recipes to help get you to the other side:

- Eat little and often to keep your blood sugar stable as low blood sugar can make you feel weak, dizzy and even faint.
- Try to stay one step ahead of the nausea. Plant a snack next to your bed so you can eat it as soon as you wake up (or in the middle of the night).
- Rest or nap whenever you can to keep your energy reserves up.
- Suck ice cubes, ice lollies or frozen watermelon and orange segments.
- Eat something nice and filling before you go to bed: a warm bowl of porridge or some cereal.
- Ginger and fennel have been used for centuries to settle the stomach. Chew fennel seeds or add chopped ginger to warm water with lemon.
- Keep it simple and carb-heavy: plain mash, dry toast, crackers, rice cakes.
- Try to up your zinc intake: walnuts, pumpkin seeds, oatmeal, cashews, wholemeal bread, eggs, red meat.
- Have mints with you at all times.
- Sniff lemons.
- Acupuncture can help, or try acupressure wristbands.
- Eat what you can. Now is not the time to beat yourself up over family-sized packs of salt-and-vinegar chipsticks for breakfast. Needs must and all that.
- If you really can't stomach the thought of food, make sure you keep sipping water to stay hydrated and stave off hyperemesis (see page 19).

QUICK AND SIMPLE RECIPES

TOPPINGS 3 WAYS

Sliced **avocado** and a **hard-boiled egg**.

Half an **apple**, sliced, spread with a couple of teaspoons of **cashew butter**.

1–2 tablespoons **hummus** with **cucumber** sprinkled with **pumpkin seeds**.

ROASTED TOMATO AND RED PEPPER SOUP

FULL OF VITAMIN C, LYCOPENE, B6, MAGNESIUM

AND ANTIOXIDANTS

Method: Chop 6 large **tomatoes**, 1 **white onion** and 1 **red pepper** into big chunks. Generously cover with **olive oil** and roast at 200°C (180°C fan oven) for 30–45 minutes or until the edges start to blacken. Remove from the oven and put in saucepan. Add 500 ml **vegetable stock**, then stir in **basil** until it wilts. Blitz with a hand-held blender. Season and serve.

ENERGY BOMBS

CONTAIN ESSENTIAL FATTY ACIDS, FIBRE, FOLATE,

VITAMIN E, IRON AND POTASSIUM

Pop them in your bag, stash them next to your bed, pile them up in the fridge. Or, for best results, do what I do and freeze them – they melt in the mouth. Method: Blitz 100g **pecans** with a cup of **oats**, then add in 2 **medjool dates**, 2 tbsps **coconut oil** and 1 tbsp **cashew butter**. Roll into balls and dust with **shredded coconut**. Freeze for best results – they defrost in seconds.

TIPS FROM MUMS:

'I ate anything ginger-flavoured – the teabags were particularly good and the ginger crystal chews. I don't know whether it really helped – maybe it was just psychological – but needless to say I can't stand the smell or taste of it now!'

'I only wanted savoury foods and found peanut butter on rice cakes really helpful, especially to take into work for a snack at my desk. It seemed to help sickness mid-morning once my breakfast had been digested.'

'My sickness was mainly in the evening, so I just ate a small meal and went straight to bed. Not very sociable for my poor husband, though!'

'I wore travel-sickness bands that you wear on your wrist and a small button pushes on a certain acupressure point. The only problem is if you're trying not to tell anyone you're pregnant you'll have to wear long-sleeve tops so as not to show the bands. But they really seemed to help.'

I was one of the lucky few who hadn't experienced any morning sickness and prided myself on the fact. Fifteen weeks into my pregnancy my partner and I treated ourselves with a trip to Barcelona to see in the New Year. When we landed I started to feel a bit dodgy but put it down to the flight, but on board the bus to the hotel a wave of dizziness and heat washed over me. Before we had a chance to escape I opened my handbag and threw up inside it. We made a quick exit with a bag full of sick and didn't look back. I spent the rest of the weekend airing out my bag and hanging my head in shame. I never boasted about anything pregnancy-related again!

Rochelle, mum of one

I KNEW I WAS PREGNANT BECAUSE I COULDN'T FIT INTO MY BRA

It's amazing how early on your body gives you signs that you might be pregnant. Women often give me a whole range of reasons for how they just 'knew' that they were pregnant, even before taking a pregnancy test. And one of the most common early pregnancy symptoms is changes to your boobs. You may notice tenderness around that area, especially if anyone tries to touch them, or a tingling sensation around the nipple. So sorry to your partner, but no chance of a quick fondle tonight; these puppies are a no-go area. It can feel a bit like an exaggerated version of how your boobs feel before a period and some women find they have to sleep in a sports bra at night as it's painful to lie on their front. Whatever your experience, when it comes to your boobs, it's important to start thinking about their important role in pregnancy and beyond.

Extra blood flow in your body caused by the hormone oestrogen makes your breast tissue swell, so don't be surprised if you go up a cup size in the first 12 weeks of pregnancy. Other changes to your boobs include increased visibility of blue veins, a darkened areola (the round bit of tissue your nipple sits on) and more prominent nipples. During pregnancy you will have up to 50 per cent more blood volume in your body, hence why your breasts may resemble an aerial photo of London. As your ribcage expands to make room for the baby, you may find that you need a bigger back size too. So don't have a breakdown when the lady says you've gone up from a 32B to a 36B. You won't have a broad back for ever, promise.

If your boobs do go through a period of rapid growth, you may find that they feel itchy as the skin stretches. Try not to scratch them too much, as that

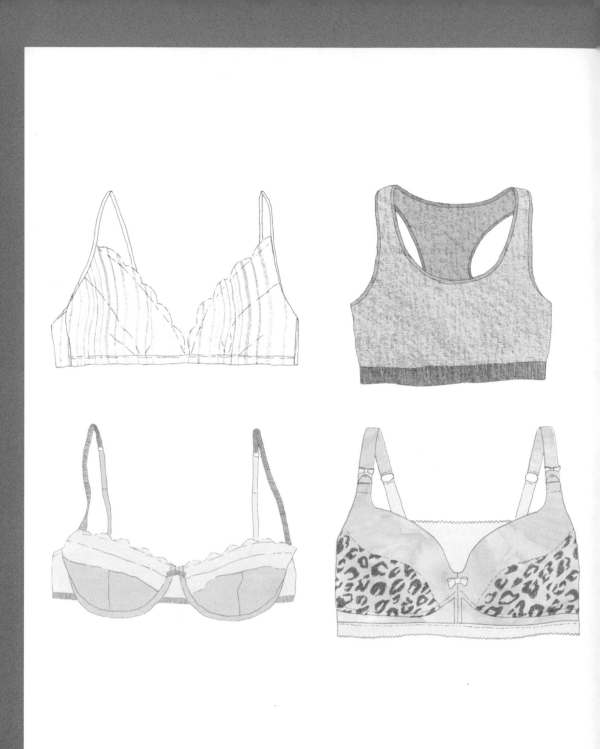

can leave horrible red marks, which can become sore. The best thing to do is to invest in a lovely pregnancy moisturiser to leave you smelling gorgeous. It's never too early in your pregnancy to start looking after your skin.

It's also worth remembering that this feeling of tenderness/soreness/don't EVEN try to touch them won't last for ever. Usually, once the hormones have done their super-amazing bit in early pregnancy, i.e. keeping that tiny bean alive and kick-starting the functions of the placenta, things should calm down.

My body didn't seem to get the memo in puberty about boobs – I was always so flat-chested the boys at school called me pancake tits. So when I became pregnant my once non-existent chest started to grow, and I could finally wear bras that were a 32B! I felt womanly and sexy for the first time in my life. God bless pregnancy hormones.

Becky, mum of one

As your regular bras are not designed to provide the support and comfort you need as your boobs grow heavier and become more sensitive, you need to think about getting fitted for new bras for your pregnancy. You may find you have growth spurts throughout the 9 months, so it's important to get measured at least twice while you're pregnant to ensure you're wearing the right size bra. I recommend getting measured at around 12–15 weeks and again at 34 weeks. Most high-street department stores offer a free measuring and fitting service and can guide you as to which bra is best for your shape. Maternity bras are designed to accommodate your changing shape, your expanding ribcage, and the increased strain on your chest muscles. As an added bonus, when maternity bras are worn regularly, they can help prevent stretch marks because they provide the right kind of support. Yay! You can also save money by buying maternity bras that can be used as nursing bras too. Double bonus. So remember, ladies: invest in your breasts!

MIDWIVES ARE VAMPIRES!

You may never have had a blood test before and suddenly you're pregnant and we want your blood! There are numerous routine blood tests offered to you that your midwife will explain about at your booking appointment. They are important, providing us with vital information about you while we care for you. It may seem like a lot of blood when you see all the bottles (usually five), but just one prick of the needle will fill the lot. Midwives are used to taking blood on a daily basis, though, so the good news is we're highly skilled at doing it – so it's quick and painless for you. If you're a bit funny about having blood taken, there's no better time to start overcoming these feelings because you'll be offered more blood tests at the 12-week scan and later at 28 weeks (see pages 29–31). It's a good idea to eat something prior to the booking appointment and have some water handy.

All of these blood tests are optional, so of course you can decline. Think carefully about why you wouldn't want to have them, though. I know it can feel a bit overwhelming with all the screening tests you are offered at your booking appointment, so take the time to read all the information leaflets your midwife gives you. Ask questions and make sure you understand the explanations given to you so you are making an informed choice.

So what are all these tests for?
- Blood group. It's important to know your blood group in the unlikely event you need a blood transfusion during pregnancy or birth. Blood group O is the most common. Groups A, B and AB are less so. You may already know your blood group, especially if you have donated blood, but we still need to have it on your hospital notes.

- Rhesus factor. If you're rhesus positive (RhD positive), you have a particular protein on the surface of your red blood cells. If you're rhesus negative

(RhD negative), you don't. If you're RhD negative and the father of your baby is positive, there's a good chance your baby will be RhD positive, too. In this case, if some of your baby's blood enters your bloodstream, your immune system may react to the D antigen in your baby's blood. It will be treated as a foreign invader and your body will produce antibodies to defend against it. In order to prevent this from happening you will be offered an injection of Anti D or immunoglobulin at 28 weeks. If you have any bleeding in pregnancy, it may also be recommended that you have an additional dose of Anti D as well as the routine one at 28 weeks. So if you go into hospital with bleeding always make sure you tell the midwife or doctor that your blood group is RhD negative. If your partner knows he is also RhD Negative you do not have the Anti D injection.

- Iron levels. A blood test can tell you if your haemoglobin levels are low, which is a sign of iron-deficiency anaemia. Your body needs around 14.8mg of iron per day to produce haemoglobin to carry oxygen around the body in your red blood cells. This keeps you feeling well, alert and not low in energy. If you're anaemic due to iron deficiency, you need to think about the best foods to eat to boost your iron stores. Think Popeye: spinach, red meat, chicken, wholegrains (see pages 44–5). You will be able to have your haemoglobin levels checked again at 28 weeks (see page 76). *I know my haemoglobin levels are always a bit low but iron tablets make me constipated. What else can I try?*
There are other options available if you choose not to take iron tablets. Products such as Floradix and Spatone are great alternative options, available from all major health-food shops. Remember that iron is absorbed better with vitamin C, so take this with a glass of fresh orange juice for an extra boost.

- Hepatitis B. You could be a carrier of the hepatitis B virus and not even know it. A blood test is often the only way to find out for certain. If you pass the disease on to your baby either before or after he or she is born, his or her liver could be seriously damaged. Babies at risk of catching hepatitis B virus from their mums can be protected with a vaccination and antibodies, given as soon as they're born.

- Syphilis. This sexually transmitted disease is fairly rare nowadays. However, if you have it and it isn't treated during pregnancy, it could cause abnormalities in your baby. Syphilis can even cause a baby to be stillborn. It is easily treated with penicillin.

- HIV/AIDS. All pregnant women are offered a blood test to detect HIV and AIDS, but you can decline if you want to. If you discover you have the infection, steps can be taken to almost eliminate the chance of the virus being transmitted to your baby during pregnancy, birth and afterwards.

GROUP B STREP

Group B strep is a normal and healthy bacteria that lives naturally in the gut flora in about 20 per cent of women. It is usually harmless, although it can pose a risk to your baby if it is passed on during childbirth. The NHS don't routinely test for Group B strep unless you have had an infection like a UTI (urine infection) or require a vaginal swab in pregnancy. For more information speak to your midwife.

12-WEEK SCAN: WHAT TO EXPECT

The 12-week scan, or nuchal translucency scan, is organised by your midwife or GP to take place between 11 and 14 weeks and it is usually performed at the hospital at which you are 'booked'. If everything in your pregnancy has gone smoothly up until now, this will be your first scan and the first glimpse of your baby and his or her little beating heart as well as a few somersaults – if you're lucky! As well as this, your baby will be measured and the approximate date that you will deliver will be calculated (EDD or estimated delivery date). This date is more accurate than the one worked out from your last menstrual period or LMP, so it is better to stick to this, although bear in mind that the majority of women do NOT deliver exactly on time.

You will also be offered screening to assess the risk of certain chromosomal disorders that may affect your pregnancy. If you choose to undergo this then the back of your baby's neck will also be measured (nuchal translucency) and this combined with a blood test will be used to assess your risk (see below).

What happens during the scan?
The scan is usually performed by a sonographer (person trained in scanning) or a doctor. Often in bigger hospitals there may be more than one person present, particularly if someone is being trained, so don't be too surprised if there is more of an audience than you'd expected! If this is the case then be prepared for the scan to take a little longer. Some women enjoy this as they get to see their baby for longer and often also get more pictures as the trainees are so grateful for your patience! However, if this does not appeal to you, please say so as it's important that you feel comfortable with what's going on.

To begin the scan you will be asked to lie down on a couch and expose your tummy area. Scanning gel (often very cold!) will be applied to your tummy and a probe will be used to see your pregnancy. Don't be too alarmed if the sonographer or doctor stops being so chatty at this point as it can take a bit of concentration to orientate themselves in your womb. Once they have a good view they will show you your baby and point out the flickering of its heartbeat before performing the rest of the scan. This usually involves a survey of the rest of your womb to confirm how many babies there are and to check that the spine, limbs and organs are all developing well. They won't, however, be able to tell you the baby's sex as it's a little early. If you do wish to find out, then this is usually offered at the 20-week scan (although bear in mind that identifying the sex via a scan is not 100 per cent accurate. They will then measure the back of the baby's neck as part of the combined test to assess risk of chromosomal disorders.

At the end of your scan, you will be given a copy of the report to put in your hand-held notes and your risk of chromosomal disorders will be explained to you. In some cases the results may not be available immediately and will therefore be sent to you in the post with an explanation of what they mean and if any further tests are needed. You will also be given a chance to buy some pictures of your baby, but costs vary from hospital to hospital.

So, what are these chromosomal abnormalities?

Chromosomes are the units that contain our genetic material. Most humans have 46 chromosomes or 23 pairs of chromosomes. Chromosomal abnormalities occur when a baby has extra chromosomes that give rise to syndromes causing different disabilities. The chromosomal abnormalities that are looked for are called Down's (or trisomy 21, so three copies instead of two copies of the 21st chromosome), Patau's (or trisomy 13, an extra copy of the 13th chromosome) and Edwards' syndromes (or trisomy 18, an extra copy of the 18th chromosome). The majority of these cases occur spontaneously, i.e., are NOT inherited, although the risk of your pregnancy being affected does increase with age.

The risk to your pregnancy is calculated using the measurement of the back of your baby's neck combined with the results of a blood test. The majority of women are found to be low-risk; however, please remember that this is a screening test, so even if your risk comes back as a 1-in-a-million chance, that still does not mean that there isn't any chance of your pregnancy being affected.

If your risk is greater than 1 in 150, then you will be offered more testing. This is usually in the form of an amniocentesis, which involves taking a sample of the fluid surrounding your baby to confirm whether he or she is affected or not. If this is recommended to you, then it will probably be done at a later date, which often gives you time to process the information as it can be a lot to take in at once. Remember that 1 in 150 is still less than a 1 per cent chance of your baby being affected, but understandably women often still want further testing to know what is happening with their baby and to guide their future decisions about the pregnancy.

The dating scan is an exciting experience and is usually the first time you will actually get to see the baby growing inside of you and start to feel that your pregnancy is actually real. It can also be a scary, anxious time, filled with anticipation, often with lots of things going on which you may not have time to process. Try to enjoy the experience and remember, the sonographer or doctor performing the scan is there for you, to explain things – so if there is anything you want to know or don't understand, please ask!

Sukhera Furness, obstetrician

GETTING THROUGH THE WORK CHRISTMAS PARTY

Without a doubt there will be the dreaded invitation to that party, wedding or work event that you just can't face attending at this stage of pregnancy. However, you may still be keeping this pregnancy a secret until you've had your 12-week scan, so what do you do?!

I remember feeling as if the entire world was having BBQs, endless engagement parties and, of course, weddings the summer I found out I was pregnant. Some events we managed to avoid due to 'other commitments', but the big ones, like our friends' weddings, were near-impossible to avoid. My husband saw it as a perfect opportunity to get absolutely wasted, with me, of course, as designated driver. Joy. So how do you manage to not get drunk but appear drunk, especially when you're feeling tired and nauseous too?

- Firstly (depending on your changing shape), choose your outfit wisely. I wasn't showing around my stomach area at 10 weeks, but my boobs were massive, so I went for a dress that didn't show my growing cleavage but was comfortable. If I had worn a maternity-style dress I think it would have made me look more pregnant than I was and a lot of friends might have become suspicious.
- Don't overdo the 'oh I'm not drinking because I'm on antibiotics/driving/ on a detox' story. It doesn't work and draws more attention to you and the situation. Take a glass of bubbles and always make sure you have an alcoholic-looking drink in your hand.
- If you're ordering drinks at the bar, try to get your trusty partner to get yours and order one that can be passed off as a gin and tonic. I'm sure there are hundreds of bartenders who have been asked to make a lemonade look like a G&T by putting it in a shorter glass and adding a slice of lime.
- Don't forget to eat! Go for the nibbles/canapés provided (but be careful of anything that might have been prepared hours before, especially meat, fish

and soft cheese). The food will keep your energy up as you won't have the buzz that alcohol gives you at these long events, and hopefully keep any waves of nausea at bay.

- Remember that the more the event goes on, the more drunk your friends will become, and the less likely they will be to notice that you're stone-cold sober. It's quite hard to act drunk when you're sober (unless you're a great actress), but be prepared for some sober dancing. Again, this is really hard because you're feeling self-conscious and you're beginning to flag, but everyone else will be having a great time, so try to manage a few obligatory wedding-dance moves to cheesy tunes.
- Make a plan with your partner on when you want to leave by; that way there won't be a big discussion in front of friends when he's having a great time and you're ready for your bed. Set a time beforehand. Make the departure very brief, i.e. only say bye to the hosts/bride and groom. That way there's less chance your friends will notice you're leaving earlier than anyone else.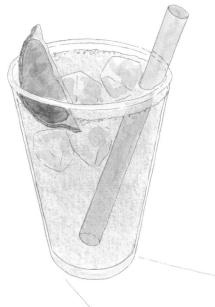
- And you can be pretty sure your partner will be feeling a million times worse than you the next day. Win–win!

TOP TIPS FOR PARTNERS

SIMON HOOPER, @FATHER_OF_DAUGHTERS

Not many people are really ever 'ready' to be parents even if it is planned, so you need to start dealing with this life-changing event sooner rather than later. If you're anything like me, then at this point in time you'll be excited but also worrying about how this is going to impact your life. Can I still go out with my friends this week? Will that special item I've been saving up for that I've wanted for ages have to go on hold in order to pay for the new pram? Will I have to get rid of my current car and replace it with something 'more practical'? Am I capable of looking after a little human? You're not alone. Mum-to-be is probably thinking about all that stuff too.

1 Talk to each other. The important thing here is that you both talk about your worries and anxieties. You're both probably feeling lots of the same things, although all those pregnancy hormones can make everything seem more overwhelming for your partner. Be there for each other — remember that you're in this together.

2 Avoid arguments. All those hormones may also mean you are sometimes the focal point of pregnancy outbursts. Defuse the situation before it erupts since stress and anger aren't good for either of you (but especially her and the baby). Suck it up/bite your tongue/take it on the chin.

3 Phone a friend. You may have friends who already have kids. If you do, then you have a ready-made support network of people who have done this before you. Ask them for advice about things you're not sure about. Men aren't always that great at talking about the touchy-feely things, but if you can move past the initial awkwardness, then you may be surprised about how good it can feel to share frustrations and worries with someone other than that special lady in your life.

4   Be there when it counts. Try to make every effort to go to antenatal checks with your partner. Hearing the heartbeat of your baby or seeing it on the scan for the first time is truly amazing. Experiencing this together will help you to bond and make the fact that you're having a baby seem so much more real. Having your support will make her feel more at ease. You won't understand all that happens in these checks, so ask some questions. Standard ones to cover (while looking at the screen and holding your partner's hand):
    • So what position are they in?
    • What are the different colours on the screen?
    • What size is the baby?

5   Stop being lazy. You may not be a culinary genius, but I'm sure you have the ability to follow a recipe from one of those 20 or so beautifully shot cookery books that adorn your kitchen shelves. So cook some nutritious meals for both of you on a weekly basis.
    I'm not saying that you should become a personal maid, but doing a bit more around the house is going to have several benefits
    • You can prove that you're capable of maintaining the house
    • She doesn't have to get stressed out about the state of the house
    • She can't have a go at you for not doing anything to help
    Note: You should expect to be told that you haven't done things to her standards and you may still get a talking-to. At this point I refer you back to point 2.

6   Read all about it. Swot up on what her body is going through. You don't have to study for a PhD but to know a little more than you do right now is no bad thing.

7   Be a team. She's going to be making some lifestyle changes over the coming months and you need to support her in them. And by support I mean make those changes too.

If you manage to do all this, I assure you that your life will be easier and it will help you mentally prepare for your new life as a parent.

18 WEEKS

IS THERE EVEN ANYTHING IN THERE?

YOUR BABY IS ABOUT THE SIZE OF AN ARTICHOKE.
IT IS A LITTLE OVER 14CM LONG AND WEIGHS ABOUT 190G

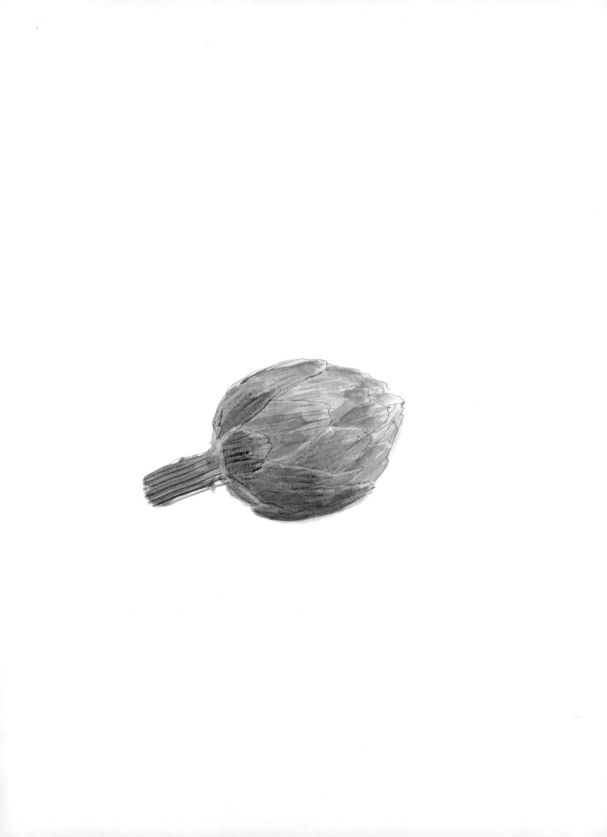

16–18 WEEKS

You made it past the worst bit of pregnancy! I really hope by the time you're reading this the nausea has gone and you've got your energy levels back. There really is nothing worse than those early weeks. Growing tiny humans is hard work, lady, and you rule! This part of your pregnancy is also called the second trimester or the 'honeymoon' period because, fingers crossed, you start to feel relatively normal, with some women even feeling at their best!

Never underestimate how much extra rest you still need from now up until you give birth; take advantage of those quiet moments when you could catch a few winks, even if it's just for 20 minutes. Getting into the habit of power-napping now is a great way to teach your body and mind how to do it when your baby is here. You'll get told by a million different people about how hard the sleep deprivation is, but one huge tip is to take daytime power-naps where possible. Babies seem to have the habit of waking lots at night for feeds and sleeping for longer periods by day (which, by the way, is totally normal for their development). So grabbing an afternoon nap when you can now will mean you're a pro when it comes to the early days. Winning!

This stage can sometimes feel as if nothing really happens. You won't have seen your midwife since your booking appointment, which must feel like a lifetime ago, but you'll be due to see them for a follow-up check by 18 weeks. At this appointment, your urine will be checked for protein, your blood pressure will be checked and, most excitingly, your midwife will be able to hear your baby's heartbeat for the first time with a small device called a sonicaid. The heartbeat can range from 110 to 160 beats per minute, but at this stage in pregnancy it will most likely be in the higher end of this range. Your midwife will reassure you what's normal. It's not recommended that you buy or use a home Doppler device to listen to your baby's heartbeat. The Kicks Count charity give the following advice to expectant parents:

It is vital that medical intervention is sought when the baby still has a heartbeat in all incidences of reduced fetal movement. So if you have any concerns about your baby's movements contact your midwife, do not rely on a home doppler. Assuming the home doppler is being used properly and is not picking up the mother's heartbeat or the placenta, the presence of a heartbeat does not indicate the baby is well. Any interventions that could save a baby in distress would need to be done when the baby has a heartbeat; leaving it until there is no heartbeat is too late.

You may have heard of all sorts of old wives' tales about the rate of your baby's heartbeat. If it sounds like a train, it's a boy, if it sounds like galloping horses, it's a girl. Both are incorrect: how can the rate at which your baby's heart beats tell you its gender? The heart rate is determined by what your baby is doing at that moment. Think about it: if the baby is very active its heart rate speeds up; if it's slower your baby is probably having a snooze. So don't use these 'theories' apart from maybe as a bit of a fun guessing game between you and your partner. The only reliable way to find out the sex of your baby is by a scan or waiting until he or she arrives!

SHOULD YOU FIND OUT THE SEX?

Probably the most commonly asked question when pregnant is 'are you going to find out the sex of the baby at the 20-week scan?' (Followed by 'when are you due?' – remember to add a week on to your estimated due date – see page 12.)

Despite being a slightly irritating question, no matter how well intended, it will be asked by everyone from your friends to your mother-in-law and the person on the checkout at the supermarket. You and your partner need to have a serious chat and decide, well, are you? It is a question that divides couples across the globe. And, of course, there are advantages and disadvantages to each argument: pros and cons that – if you're not careful – you can end up arguing about until you're blue (or pink) in the face.

There's no right or wrong answer – it's a choice that each couple has to decide on – but ideally think about it before the 20-week scan, unless you want an argument with a sonographer present, which could be awkward . . .

I've spoken to lots of women – and men – on this matter and have come up with a list of the most popular pros and cons of finding out. This list won't necessarily give you the answer – it is such a personal decision, and it has to be right for you – but if you're undecided it might give you some things for you and your partner to think about.

Remember, once you find out and the sonographer utters those words 'boy' or 'girl' there's no going back. However, there is always that very small chance that the scan isn't accurate, so don't go crazy and paint the nursery pink just in case she turns out to be a he! Also, some hospitals have a policy not to tell women the gender of their baby – so find out if yours does or not.

PROS

- You can focus your name-deciding on one gender (potentially saving hours of tedious debating).
- You can decorate the nursery in more gender-specific colours rather than sticking to the various shades of white or yellow.
- And the same goes for baby clothes.
- If this is your second baby you can help your older child prepare for a sibling. It also helps you decide whether you need to buy a new set of clothes or can just use hand-me-downs.
- Some couples say they felt closer and bonded to their unborn baby knowing the gender before birth, calling it 'he' or 'she' rather than 'it'.
- Friends and family have more direction when deciding on a gift.
- Avoids any element of disappointment if you had your heart set on a boy or a girl.

CONS

- Why spoil one of life's greatest surprises?
- Some women say it gave them an increased incentive during labour.
- It will not make you love your child any more.
- Does it really matter? As long as it's healthy.
- Finding out the gender is not 100 per cent accurate.
- Buying neutral-coloured clothes means you can use them for future sons or daughters, thus saving money.

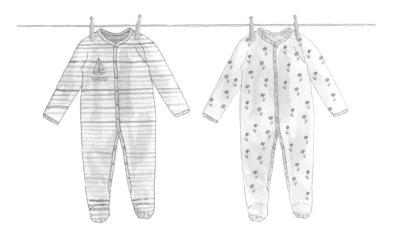

WHAT IS A DOULA?

BECCY HANDS, UK DOULA

Personal support from a close female friend or relative throughout pregnancy, labour and the post-partum period is a tradition shared by many cultures over thousands of years. In today's busy world, not everyone has such a support network, and with maternity services being cut constantly, mums-to-be are left wanting more women-centred, nurturing care. This is how doulas came to be.

A doula is experienced and trained to support a mum during pregnancy, labour and beyond, and can fill the gaps in busy maternity services by providing continual support to the woman and her partner throughout the childbearing year. A doula does not replace the midwife and medical staff, but aims to work alongside them in harmony. Neither does she replace the birth partner; instead, she will provide support so that they can focus on loving and encouraging you appropriately. If there will not be a birth partner present then a doula will fill that role too, helping you to gather information about the options available to you for birth and afterwards.

During your labour, your doula will be a constant, calming presence to guide and support you through the birth. Ideally, you will feel unobserved but very well cared for, creating the optimum conditions for a healthy labour.

Every couple and every woman is different, with their own ideas about their 'perfect birth'. It is a doula's job to get to know you and your partner, and to support whatever your vision is. This is achieved by:
- Meeting a few times before the birth/getting to know you and your wishes.
- Examining issues from previous labours/settling first-time nerves.
- Talking through the stages of labour and what to expect.
- Discussing techniques to help you cope with the birth itself.
- Helping you to write a birth plan.
- Helping pack your hospital bag, or make a list of what you need for a home birth.

During the birth your doula is an extra pair of hands to help with anything that needs doing – filling the pool, making tea, having a tidy-up, massaging your back, entertaining the kids – you name it, they can do it! They are there to support mother and birth partner with calming words, helpful suggestions to keep you comfortable, and reminders of what a fantastic job you are doing. Your doula will join you at whatever part of the labour you'd like her to – early on or later into it – and will stay with you until your baby Is born, you have had a shower and the baby has had a feed. After this they will tuck you up in bed with some tea and toast and leave you to marvel at your baby and all that you have achieved.

Your doula will be available for questions and chats from the time of booking, and will go on call for you (available any time of day or night) from two or three weeks before your due date until your baby is born. For this reason a doula will only take one or two women a month, unless she works in a team of doulas, in which case they may take more bookings. Ask your doula how she works and pick one who suits you best.

And now for the statistics! A recent report showed that women who had the support of a doula during labour had:

- labour duration reduced by 25%
- the odds of forceps reduced by 40%
- 30% reduction in requests for pain relief
- 60% reduction in use of epidural

There are hundreds of doulas listed on **www.doula.org.uk** – you can have a read of their profiles, meet for an informal cuppa and see who you click with. The doula you feel most at ease with is the doula for you! Doulas' fees range from between £250 for a mentored doula (see the website for more details on this) up to around £2,000.

I love this quote by John H. Kennell, MD:

If a doula were a drug, it would be unethical not to use it.

GETTING YOUR DIET BACK ON TRACK

EMMA BARDWELL, HEALTH AND WELLNESS
WRITER, @EIGHTYPERCENTCLEAN

The nausea is waning. Hell, you might even be starting to glow! You've only gone and made it to your second trimester. This is allegedly the good 'middle bit' before you start dealing with piles, gargantuan nipples and uncontrollable wind. (You've got that already? Totally normal.) It's also the bit where your baby starts noticeably growing. Nutrition is the cornerstone of a healthy pregnancy, but chances are you've consumed your fair share of junk food over the last few weeks, especially if you've been suffering from morning sickness or fatigue. Here then are a few tips to get you back on track.

- Try starting the day with hot water and lemon. It's a good alternative to caffeine and jumpstarts your digestive juices.
- Focus on the quality, rather than the quantity, of food (unfortunately, the school of thought that said you should be eating for two has closed down).
- Try to make better choices, rather than perfect ones. We all know fresh, unprocessed food is best but if you accidentally inhaled a box of doughnuts for breakfast, don't beat yourself up.
- Omega-3s are your best friends and great for brain health – yours and your baby's. Find them in pumpkin seeds, hemp seeds, chia seeds, walnuts, eggs and dark leafy vegetables, as well as low-mercury fish such as sardines, mackerel and wild salmon.
- Drink lots of water. Constipation is the LAST thing you need right now.
- You're using a lot of iron to make all that extra blood for your baby. Boost your intake with green leafy veg such as spinach or kale, good-quality (preferably organic) lean meat, beans, lentils, cashews and

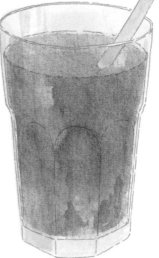

pumpkin seeds. Try a watercress and baby spinach salad with lightly fried halloumi and ripe papaya (vitamin C aids iron absorption).

- Try taking a good probiotic or add a natural source such as kefir (fermented yoghurt) to your diet. Good gut health is all-important.
- Chew your food really well and eat slowly. Heartburn and indigestion are common in pregnancy and often get worse as your growing baby starts putting the squeeze on your internal organs.
- Fill your fridge with healthy, easy-prep foods: avocados, quinoa, yoghurt, fresh berries, nori wraps, energy bombs (see page 21), eggs, salads, juices, smoothies, sweetcorn and almond butter (delicious with apple slices).

EASY BREAKFAST CHIA PUDDING
SOURCE OF PROTEIN, IRON, CALCIUM AND VITAMIN C
Mix 4 tbsps of **chia seeds** with 250ml of **almond milk**. Add a blob of **yoghurt**, a tsp of **vanilla paste**, some **desiccated coconut** and a sprinkle of **cinnamon**. Leave in the fridge overnight. In the morning add **fresh berries**, **pomegranate, nuts, goji berries, seeds, nut butter** – whatever you have.

GREEN SMOOTHIE
CONTAINS FIBRE, IRON, VITAMIN C AND E, CALCIUM, POTASSIUM, MAGNESIUM AND ZINC
Blitz a handful of **kale**, a handful of **spinach**, juice of half a **lemon**, a cup of **almond milk**, half a **pear**, half a **banana** and a tbsp of **almond butter**.

QUICK LUNCH OR SUPPER PEA AND FETA FRITTATA
FULL OF OMEGA-3, CALCIUM, FIBRE, VITAMIN D, B6, B12, FOLATE AND CHOLINE
Blitz 120g defrosted **peas** with 2 **eggs**. Fold in 30g **rice flour**. Stir in 125g chopped **red pepper** (or mushrooms or ham – whatever you have), 60g crumbled **feta**, a chopped **red chilli**, 3 chopped **spring onions**, small bunch of chopped **parsley, salt** and **pepper**. Heat a tbsp of **coconut oil** in a frying pan and spoon in a large dollop of batter; spread out with a spatula. Heat gently until it browns and firms up, then flip to cook the other side.

WIND OR BABY?

Now that you're hopefully feeling better, you're probably eagerly waiting for those first precious feelings of your baby moving in your tummy. During your 12-week scan your baby is often so active in there, the sonographer can find it hard to take the required measurements. During the scan with my twins they looked as if they were taking part in a Zumba class. But isn't it bizarre that you can't feel a single movement? It can sometimes make the whole experience very surreal and abstract: is that even my baby and my uterus? Small, gentle kicks are also known as 'quickening' and can be so subtle most first-time pregnant women brush them off as hunger pangs or wind passing through their tummy. Everyone feels their baby move at different stages: some as early as 15 weeks and some not until after the 20-week scan. There is no right and wrong here; it's based on lots of different factors.

- The number of pregnancies you've had. Most second- and third-time pregnant women report that they felt their baby move earlier, mainly due to the body knowing and recognising those feelings as baby and not wind.
- Where the placenta is positioned. At your 12-week scan the sonographer will have detected your placenta and said whether it was anterior (at the front of your uterus) or posterior (at the back of your uterus). If you have an anterior placenta the initial kicks may not feel as strong in the early stages as your baby has a big fat squidgy cushion to kick against.
- Your physique. We are all designed differently and come in all shapes and sizes – some of us are blessed with toned washboard stomachs, some are more like me – a little loose and wobbly around that area. Very slim women do seem to be able to feel those first flutters earlier.
- What you're doing. If you're busy at work or rushing about you're not going to feel those subtle movements, which is why lots of women say they first felt them when they were lying still in the bath or in bed at night.

Over the next few weeks it is a good idea to make a note of your baby's activity pattern. Do they kick more in the morning or evening? Do they have spells when they make a lot of movements? This will help you determine if there is a change in your baby's regular pattern of movement. You won't necessarily feel these kicks every day at this stage: it doesn't mean your baby isn't moving lots inside because it definitely will be, it's just that the movements are so small and subtle. As your baby grows and gets stronger the movements will feel stronger; much more like proper kicks rather than flutters or pops. And remember to try not to compare yourself with your pregnant friends – like I said, everyone is different and that includes your baby.

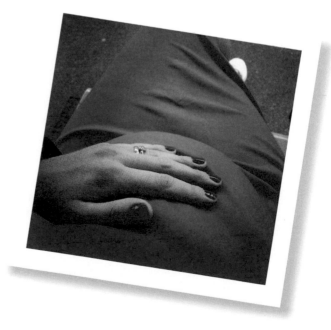

PILATES IN PREGNANCY

ANYA JOELI, PILATES TEACHER

Make sure you attend a class that is suitable for pregnancy.

1 Your baby uses your pelvic floor as a trampoline for a good few months, so you need it to be in top working order. All Pilates exercises focus on pelvic-floor awareness and strength.

2 You'll also need to be able to release your pelvic floor to allow your baby to exit. Pregnancy Pilates teaches you to fully relax 'down there', being mindful of your body and its tensions.

3 Your abdominals stretch as your bump grows, and in most pregnancies they actually split down the middle; this is called diastasis recti. Pilates builds an extra corset of strength to support your back and bump, and to ensure they zip back up once your baby is no longer in your belly.

4 Pilates corrects your posture. Do you slump in your seat? Pilates irons you out to ensure you cope well with the added load of your growing baby.

5 Breath influences and indicates our state of mind and well-being. Pilates encourages you to breathe fully and deeply, which aids relaxation, and is also an effective tool during labour.

6 Pilates is perfect for relieving tension and anxiety. By connecting to your body and achieving balance, you can also release your mind.

7 You can practise Pilates during labour: Pilates squats allow the pelvis to widen to help your baby descend. Regular practice means during labour you'll be able to enter a familiar physical state and get into a 'zone'.

8 You'll tone the bits of your body that don't have as good an excuse to balloon – your arms, thighs, bum…

9 It's a safe way to stretch and move your body through all trimesters.

10 Pilates limits the challenges that pregnancy places on your body, and gives you some space to become more in tune with your body.

PREGNANCY YOGA

TAMMY MITTELL, YOGA TEACHER

Pregnancy and yoga are highly compatible because yoga is a tool to explore the depths of our human nature and there is nothing more natural than having a baby. In pregnancy, a woman's senses are heightened: she can smell more vividly and is more sensitive to taste and to emotional states. This is because she becomes more intuitive. Practising yoga will help tune into those intuitions to positively experience the transformation into motherhood. The breathing techniques, gentle movement exercises, meditation and relaxation methods provide practical tools to support a woman on her journey through pregnancy, labour, post-natal recovery and well into motherhood. Benefits include:

1 Keeps the body supple without strain and helps maintain balance as your centre of gravity changes.
2 Builds strength and stamina while maintaining joint stability.
3 Brings awareness to, and enhances, the tone of the pelvic floor for labour and better post-natal recovery.
4 Relieves common minor ailments during pregnancy, e.g. swollen joints – fat ankles, heartburn, constipation, hip and lower back pain.
5 Prevents stretch marks by increasing the elasticity of the skin.
6 Boosts energy and combats exhaustion.
7 Grounding and centring practice relieves anxiety and calms emotional turbulence, promoting relaxation and restful sleep.
8 Breath awareness and control along with visual techniques help manage contractions during labour.
9 Lots of all-four poses – said to help with optimal fetal positioning.
10 Cultivates core strength safely, to help close abdominal diastasis postnatally.

THE 20-WEEK, OR ANOMALY, SCAN

DR SURABHI NANDA

In the majority of women, the 20-week scan, which is also known as the 'anomaly scan', would be the second time they would see their baby, the first scan being around 12 weeks. The anomaly scan is offered in most units between weeks 18 and 20 of pregnancy, although some units may offer it a bit later, up to 23 weeks. This later scan is offered in units where there are extra screening tests available as a part of research for predicting risk of developing high blood pressure or having a small baby in that pregnancy. The anomaly scan is offered to all pregnant women, and there should be written information about it provided by the midwife earlier in pregnancy.

The main purpose of the anomaly scan is to check that the baby is developing normally, rather than checking the gender of the baby. The gender, however, may be disclosed following the scan, upon request, although some hospitals have a policy of not telling parents-to-be. The person carrying out the scan is usually a sonographer who is trained in providing this service to the specific standards that are expected of this scan by the NHS Fetal Anomaly Screening Programme (FASP). It is, however, important that each woman attending the scan has realistic expectations of the process and its outcomes.

During the scan, various parts of the baby's body are checked to look for any abnormality, 'defects' or 'malformations'. The sonographer looks at the shape and structure of the baby's head to check for brain or skull defects; the face, to check for a cleft lip and sometimes a cleft palate, which is usually hard to see and often not picked up; the baby's spine, to make sure that all the bones align, and that the skin covers the spine at the back, which will help indicate whether a condition called spina bifida is present. In addition, a detailed assessment of the baby's heart is carried out as per the guidance laid out by the Fetal Anomaly Screening Programme. The baby's abdominal wall (future belly button) is checked to ensure it covers all the internal organs. The baby's kidneys, bladder, stomach, swallowing and movements are checked. The sonographer will look at the baby's fingers and toes, but not count them. The baby is then measured, based on the head, tummy (at the level of the waist) and thigh bone to get an estimated weight. This, however, does not reflect the weight of the baby at birth. To ensure that the baby is growing normally, regular visits to the midwife are recommended and an additional scan in late pregnancy is offered if there are any concerns. It is not possible to measure the length of the baby on this scan. The anomaly scan also checks the position of the placenta, and if the placenta is lying low in the womb (uterus), an additional scan is offered late in the pregnancy. The anomaly scan does not usually offer 3D/4D pictures of the baby.

Sometimes, despite best efforts, the scan cannot be completed at the first appointment. Factors limiting the quality of the scan may be the position of the fetus, presence of extra tummy fat, bloating, scar tissue or fibroids, or increased or decreased water around the baby. In such cases, an additional scan is offered around 23 weeks. If there is an 'anomaly' detected on the scan, the sonographer will arrange a referral for a specialist fetal medicine scan within three to five working days.

As far as we know, the baby is unaware that the scan is taking place and this scan is not thought to be harmful to the mother or the baby. The anomaly scan is usually a pleasant experience and also serves as a bonding exercise for the expectant mother and the family. Exclamations voiced during scanning such as 'it's a baby' or 'it's surreal' – are not uncommon.

THE ANOMALY SCAN

LIZZIE, MUM OF TWO

I lay on the bed, pulled my waistband down, tucked some tissue in and the sonographer applied the gel to my tummy – whoever invented the gel-warmer is one of my favourite people in the world! Our sonographer was extremely calm, warm and professional, which helped me to relax. The first thing she said was, 'There's baby – with an excellent strong heartbeat,' which was hugely reassuring. She started the check-up with the brain and was very methodical, explaining exactly what she was looking at, measuring and why, and letting us know that things were fine before moving on.

It's completely amazing, being taken on a guided tour of this little person you've yet to meet, although my mind wandered sometimes – when the image on the screen just looked like a photocopier malfunction to the untrained eye. In those moments, especially when it seemed that all was well, I tried to decide whether or not to find out the sex – we still hadn't decided – finally picturing the birth and determining that I'd leave it a surprise.

There were also fantastic moments, like when the sonographer pointed out that the baby was yawning or turning to look at us, having a little wriggle and putting its hands up to its head in an uncanny recreation of its big sister's favourite sleeping position.

I did stress out a little bit when the sonographer said the baby's legs and feet were too curled up to assess the development and suggested we went for a walk to help it change position, saying she'd check the blood flow of the heart when we got back. She also said she wanted me to have a wee so she could have another look at the placenta after I'd emptied my bladder. Despite convincing myself that all this must mean there was a problem with the heart, legs, feet, placenta, or all of the above, the baby moved and it was absolutely fine. The sonographer also showed me my bladder, birth canal, and the location of the placenta, which is posterior, to the back of the uterus, unlike in my first pregnancy, when it was anterior, to the front, meaning I didn't feel much kicking. I've felt kicks for a few weeks already with this one, so I wasn't surprised – I even saw my stomach moving when I went to bed that night! She also checked it wasn't too low. She also spotted, accurately located and measured a small fibroid I've had for a while. This fibroid may or may not prevent me from giving birth in the hospital's birth centre, although they are currently reviewing their policy and there is an appeals system at 36 weeks for women who would like to use this facility but have, for whatever reason, been advised to have a hospital delivery.

Towards the end, I told the sonographer I didn't want to know the sex and she assured me that even she didn't know because, as we hadn't requested it, she wouldn't look.

Once she'd finished, she asked if I'd be willing for her to check the blood flow to the uterus, which is a new test the hospital is shortly bringing in for women with high blood pressure and suspected pre-eclampsia – not that I have it. I did briefly have high blood pressure towards the end of my first pregnancy, though, so I was more than happy to take part. We got to hear the roar of the blood flow on both sides of the uterus and see it represented on a graph on the screen. I asked if this was anything to do with the placenta noise that midwives pick up on their portable Doppler scanners but it's different – although apparently it sounds very similar.

By this point, I was having a whale of a time and babbling with relief! The chance to glimpse the secret world your baby inhabits for 40 weeks or so is such a terrific privilege, and I was even pretty fascinated to see my own bladder on TV! I do wish I could have been more relaxed and enjoyed the experience more but I think it's normal to be nervous. It is a serious check-up that can potentially save lives, so it's not something to be taken lightly.

Having said that, for those of us who are fortunate enough to leave clutching a batch of pictures at £3 a pop knowing everything is well, the 20-week scan is a pregnancy highlight. I've also noticed that a lot of people are waiting till this point to widely announce their pregnancy. I doubt I'll relax completely, but I now feel I can heave a big sigh of relief, break out the maternity clobber and get on with being properly pregnant.

PLUS POINTS OF BEING PREGNANT

- My liver had never had such a good detox. It must have given a huge sigh of relief that it didn't have to filter out any alcohol for almost nine months.
- And that means no hangovers. It's strangely pleasurable watching your partner suffer the day after your best friend's wedding while you joyfully skip around the kitchen offering to make bacon sarnies like the perfect wife.
- Seat on the train/tube – once my bump started to show I wore that 'Baby on Board' badge with pride.
- Excuse to buy new clothes – finding great maternity clothes on a regular basis is a great way to convince your partner you need new threads.
- (For some people) bigger boobs – it's like a free boob job on the NHS.
- An excuse to spoil yourself: if you feel like lying around in your bath robe all day, then do it!
- More melatonin in your skin means you hold on to your tan longer – I had the brownest tummy during my pregnancy.
- No periods – literally the best!
- Higher sex drive – my husband didn't know what had got into me.
- Having the best excuse not to go to stuff you really don't want to – no one will argue with the 'my back is killing and I can't stand in heels for longer than 20 minutes' reason you don't want to go to that guy from finance's leaving drinks.
- Shinier, thicker hair – you don't necessarily grow thicker hair but you lose less, which means far fewer bad-hair days. And stronger fingernails!
- Better skin – if you're one of the lucky ones. I hardly got any of those horrible teenage-spot outbreaks throughout my pregnancy and wore much less make-up than usual because my skin didn't look so tired.
- Not worrying about trying to hold your tummy in. Finally a reason to wear tight-fitting clothing; show that bump off like you mean it! Pregnancy is something to be celebrated, so be proud of your changing shape. It may

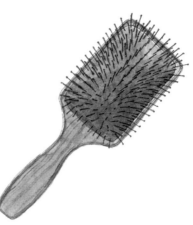

take some getting used to but
once you've nailed your pregnancy
wardrobe you'll feel a million times
better about yourself (see Zoe: Dress
like a mum, page 83).

- And finally, just feeling a bit special.
  I know women have been doing this since before history began but it's
  an incredible time in your life, even if it's your second, third or fourth
  pregnancy. Growing new life is amazing, so remember to embrace this
  magical time.

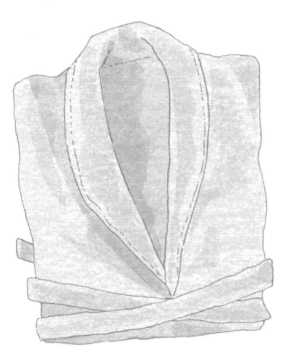

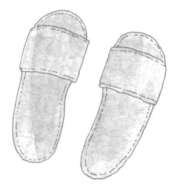

25 WEEKS

I GOT OFFERED A SEAT ON THE BUS LAST WEEK SO I MUST REALLY BE PREGNANT

YOUR BABY IS ABOUT THE SIZE OF A CAULIFLOWER.
IT IS AROUND 34.5CM LONG (FROM HEAD TO TOE, BUT
IT IS CURLED UP INSIDE YOU) AND WEIGHS ABOUT 660G.

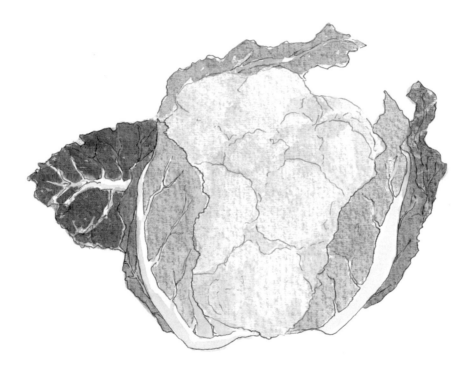

PELVIC-FLOOR EXERCISE

I always thought I had a good pelvic floor before children. I did the odd bit of exercise when I remembered, but generally I'm fit, young and healthy so 'why bother?', I thought. Throw in four babies, including a twin pregnancy, and, well, to be honest I had to do something about a potentially big problem. Seeing those adverts for women skipping through fields, so happy because they're wearing incontinence pads, made me realise I did not want to get to that stage. The good news is that pelvic-floor exercises are not like your usual workout routine. They're a simple, convenient way to get those vital muscles back into shape – no sweat! (None at all, promise.) Emma Bardwell, health and wellness writer, explains more:

First you need to find the right muscles. The best way to do this is to try to stop the flow of urine when you go to the toilet. If you can manage to do this then the muscles you used are the right ones for pelvic-floor exercises. When contracting these muscles it should feel as though you're squeezing and lifting them slightly up into the body. There shouldn't be any tensing of the buttocks or thighs, although tightening your anus can help (as if holding in wind).

- It's great to get into the practice of doing pelvic-floor exercises during your pregnancy, but really you should continue after you give birth, and beyond.
- Make sure you're activating the whole of your pelvic floor, not just the front section. The diagram shows the pelvic-floor muscles supporting all around the openings of the urethra, vagina and anus. You need to be activating all three elements of that figure-of-eight pattern, not just the front part. In pregnancy it's recommended that you do 3 sets of 8 squeezes every day; to help you remember, you could do them at each set meal time.
- Start off doing your exercises when lying down or sitting (so you're not working against gravity), then progress to standing as you improve. It's very important to completely relax your pelvic floor after each squeeze.
- Constipation is a major cause of poor bladder control and straining can

actually lead to a prolapse (when the pelvic organs drop into the path of the vagina). Keep everything moving internally with a good, clean diet made up of plenty of fruit, fibre and vegetables. If you're really struggling with constipation speak to your midwife or GP.

- Speaking of prolapses, pelvic-floor exercises can be a great first-line therapy when it comes to managing the symptoms and, in certain cases, can avoid the need for surgery.
- Train your bladder to wait longer between toilet visits. The ideal time is roughly three hours – a good wee should last around 15 seconds. Try not to go 'just in case'; it makes for a lazy bladder. Cutting down on caffeine in pregnancy is not only beneficial for your baby – it is also a diuretic.
- If you feel a cough/sneeze coming on, squeeze your pelvic-floor muscles in preparation.
- Young, old, kids in tow or not, if you're in any doubt about your pelvic-floor status quo, find a women's health physio or talk to your GP, who can refer you to a urogynaecologist. Please don't pretend it's not happening, because ignoring it won't make it go away.
- And if the last point didn't resonate, maybe this will: pelvic-floor exercises can heighten arousal during sex, give you mind-blowing orgasms, improve blood circulation and increase vaginal tone. Now you're clenching.

So come on, girls, give it a go! You don't know how much you'll miss it till it's gone, but with a bit of work you can always get it back.

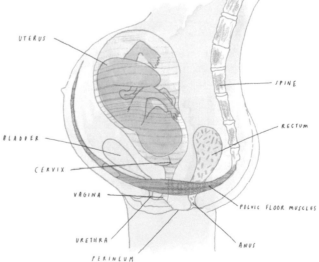

RESEARCHING THE PLACE OF BIRTH

You may think it's far too early to start entertaining the idea of giving birth – after all, your bump is only just popping out and your baby is about the size of a small cauliflower. But the earlier you start doing your research and thinking about the options available to you, the more clued up you'll be about making an informed choice. Birth is one of those emotive subjects that everyone feels they get an opinion on. If you plan a home birth you're brave (you're not brave – you're birthing with people you know in a place you know like women have done for thousands of years, and choosing a statistically safer option if you're low-risk (see page 62), as endorsed by NICE and the NHS); and if you have a caesarean you're allegedly 'too posh to push' (but interestingly, not too posh for the footless stockings and the catheter knocking around your knees in the aftermath). Just to note that in this context 'normal births' are defined as 'without induction, caesarean, instrumental delivery or episiotomy, but including epidurals and other anaesthetic.'

OPTION	PROS	CONS
Home birth A planned birth at home with a midwife providing care during labour and following birth. Midwives are trained to help you give birth at home safely, and will also advise you if transferring into an obstetric unit would be best. You can choose to give birth in or out of water – the option is available to hire or buy a birth pool.	• Less likely to have medical intervention • Less likely to use pain relief, i.e. an epidural • You may feel more comfortable labouring in your own environment • More likely to know your midwife • No evidence of difference in safety in low-risk women	• Continuous monitoring of the baby's heartbeat not possible at home • You may need to transfer into an obstetric unit should any complications arise or if you decide to have an epidural • In the unlikely event of something going wrong, the outcome for mother or baby may be worse at home than in hospital. Midwives carry the essential

The option to have the baby at home should be available to all in the UK, but further discussion with your midwife, Supervisor of Midwives or obstetrician may be recommended, depending on your pregnancy risk factors.

equipment needed for normal birth, which may not be advanced enough in a serious emergency

Midwife-led unit (freestanding) Based at a centre on a separate site from the nearest main hospital. Midwives take responsibility for your care during labour and support you to have a normal birth.	• Intervention rates are lower	• You may need to transfer into an obstetric unit should any complications arise or if you decide to have an epidural. This is more likely for first-time mothers
Midwife-led unit (alongside) Based in hospitals – separate from obstetric units. Midwives take responsibility for care during labour, and support you to have a normal birth.	• Intervention rates are lower for planned home and midwifery unit births • Should you need to transfer to an obstetric unit, it's in the same location	• You may need to transfer into an obstetric unit should any complications arise or if you decide to have an epidural
Obstetric units Based in hospitals, these units provide 24-hour services including medical, obstetric, neonatal and anaesthetic care. Although care is provided by a team of people, obstetricians lead care if you're 'high-risk'. Midwives also provide care in an obstetric unit, and lead your care if you have a straightforward pregnancy and birth.	• Should any complications arise, you're in the right place to get them addressed quickly • All drugs and equipment are available • Access to full anaesthetic services, including an epidural • Safer for women with any pre-existing medical problems	• More likely to use pain relief, e.g. opiates and epidural • Lower chance of having a normal birth • Higher chance of medical intervention including an assisted delivery and C-section

Source: Birth Place Study, NICE, RCM normal birth

WHAT IS A LOW-RISK PREGNANCY?

When thinking about where to have your baby, it is a good idea to consider where you will feel the safest and the most comfortable. And much depends on whether yours is considered a low-risk pregnancy.

A 'low-risk pregnancy' is one where a woman is not identified as having certain medical factors before going into labour. These include:

- Long-term medical conditions such as heart disease, high blood pressure, severe asthma, cystic fibrosis, diabetes and blood disorders such as sickle-cell disease.
- Infections such as HIV or hepatitis B or C, or current infection with chickenpox, German measles or genital herpes.
- Psychiatric disorders requiring current inpatient care.
- Complications with previous pregnancies.
- Complications during their current pregnancy, such as multiple births, placenta praevia (where the placenta is positioned over the cervix), pre-term labour, pre-eclampsia, onset of gestational diabetes, damage to the placenta, induction of labour, and breech position of the baby. Risks may also include a 'small for gestational age' baby, or if the baby had an abnormal fetal heart rate.
- Maternal age of over 40.

Giving birth is generally very safe wherever you choose to have your baby. If you have a low-risk pregnancy and there are no reasons why your birth may be more complicated, then there's no reason to automatically choose a hospital with the highest-of-high tech going.

If you are having your first baby, your midwife should advise you that planning birth in a midwife-led unit is suitable for you. This is because:
- The chances of your baby having a serious medical problem (which are

very low) are not affected compared with planning birth in an obstetric unit, but there is a small increase in the chance of a serious problem for your baby if you plan to give birth at home (adapted from NICE guidelines).

- You are less likely to have interventions (such as a ventouse or forceps birth, caesarean section and episiotomy) compared with giving birth in an obstetric unit.

Remember that things can change in pregnancy, so be open-minded when thinking about your options and ask your midwife for further information. The most important thing is that you choose to give birth where you are going to feel happiest and supported. See over the page for some key questions to ask your midwife.

QUESTIONS TO ASK YOUR MIDWIFE

Where you choose to give birth affects your overall experience. As a midwife I truly believe that providing you with evidence-based information helps you to make the right choices. Pregnancy and birth is unknown territory to most first-time mothers, so asking your midwife the right questions will help you and your partner feel more prepared. Here are some starter questions to help you get the most from your birth discussions:

- Am I low- or high-risk?
- What birth settings might be suitable for me?
- Is there a dedicated 'home birth' team? If so, how many midwives are on call?
- What happens if someone else is in labour at the same time?
- What pain relief is available at home?
- What about any mess at home? Do the midwives help clear up?
- In an emergency what percentage of women transfer from home to hospital during labour?
- And what reasons do you transfer in for?
- Does the local hospital have a midwife-led unit?
- If birthing pools are provided, how many pools are available to use?
- Is there a tour of the hospital for women and their birth partners?
- How many birth partners can I have with me in hospital?
- Can my partner stay overnight with me?
- What are the statistics for interventions, including C-sections?
- Is the hospital Baby Friendly Accredited? See: www.unicef.org.uk/BabyFriendly/About-Baby-Friendly/Awards/
- What sort of special care baby unit is available?
- If the birth is straightforward, how quickly can I come home?
- When do I need to decide my options by?
- Do I have to use the hospital closest to me or can I choose another one?

PLACE OF BIRTH CHECKLIST

When deciding on where you would like to give birth, it's really important that your partner is on board with your wishes. After all, he or she will be the one inflating the pool for a home birth or calling for the taxi if you decide to have a hospital birth. This checklist is a great tool to go through together.

- How do hospitals make me feel?
- Where would I feel safe and supported?
- Do I want a water birth?
- Do I want an epidural?
- Can I have a pool at home?
- How many home births do our community midwives attend per month?
- How long would it take to get to the nearest hospital in an ambulance?
- How would we feel if something didn't go to plan at home?
- Will the house get messy if we have a home birth?
- If labour starts in the middle of the night can my older child stay in bed asleep at home?
- What would I need to buy for a home birth?
- How good is the hospital in an emergency?
- What pain relief can I have at home vs hospital?

Remember it's your birth; your choice. You should never be told to do anything, but only be given choices. Every option offered to you should include benefits and risks and should be given alternatives. The good news is that you can change your mind at any time during your pregnancy, even during labour. If you have booked a hospital birth, you can decide to stay at home, or if you have booked a home birth you can decide to go to hospital. Another great tool to help you decide where you would like to have your baby is: www.which.co.uk/birth-choice.

PELVIC ACHES AND PAINS

THE WONDERS OF PREGNANCY MASSAGE

Beccy Hands (yes, that is her real surname), pregnancy massage therapist and doula, explains why women shouldn't just be putting up with 'common pregnancy aches and pains' – backache, aching hips and pelvic pain.

We are so used to hearing about pregnancy aches and pains that we don't realise that a lot of these so-called 'pregnancy ailments' can be avoided. Achy hips, pelvic girdle pain, pubis pain or sciatica, to name a few common problems, can all be helped and often stopped with massage and other body work. There are many causes of hip and pelvic aches in pregnancy, from an increase in the hormone relaxin to things as simple as having to sleep on your side, which puts pressure on the hips. Whatever the cause, a good therapist trained in treating women pre- and post-partum will know which areas to target to support the changes your body is going through. They will be able to advise on posture, show you stretches and talk you through everyday self-help tips so you can enjoy a pain-free pregnancy.

Women I see, who have regular treatments throughout pregnancy, also rarely suffer with the other ailments we commonly associate as just being 'part of pregnancy'. What better way to keep cramps, heartburn, sleepless nights, tight shoulders, painful hips and achy backs at bay than pregnancy massage? And if that wasn't reason enough to treat yourself to regular body work, then how about this: during a massage we release endorphins, the hormones that make us feel happy and relaxed. These wonderful hormones then cross through the placenta, meaning your baby enjoys the massage too.

As a society we need to encourage women to look after themselves more during pregnancy. It shouldn't be about being 'superwoman' and doing it all without making a fuss. Forget babygrows and nappy cakes, a voucher for a relaxing treatment should be top of the 'what to get an expectant mum' list!

- Most therapists advise waiting until the second trimester.
- Massage the muscles, never on the bone and keep pressure light. Build up pressure gradually, if she would like.
- Use massage oils that are safe for pregnancy and take your time – do not rush: slow repetitive strokes are best for relaxing and drainage, which can help with swollen legs, ankles, feet and hands.
- Your partner should lie on her side with a pillow under her head and one between her knees and ankles, and a blanket to keep her warm.

Back massage
The muscles on either side of the spine work hard in pregnancy and labour. Starting at the base of the spine, with a hand to either side (never on it), massage up toward the head, over the shoulders and down the sides. Repeat.

The buttocks
The buttocks can get very tight during pregnancy as they work hard to stabilise the pelvis. Using your knuckles or thumbs, press into the glutes, using little circles all over the muscle to release tension and increase lymph flow.

Hands and feet
The lymph flow around the extremities can slow down and cause fluid to pool, resulting in swelling and soreness. A hand and foot massage can relax tense muscles and encourage the pooled fluid to drain away.

The jaw
Trace the line of the jaw, pinching it gently between your thumb and finger, up toward the ear. Repeat. Next, using your finger, trace a line under the cheekbone from the nose to ear; this drains the sinus cavity and releases jaw tension. If we are tense in the jaw, we are tense in the vagina – most definitely NOT helpful in labour – think 'FLOPPY FACE, FLOPPY FANNY'.

SLEEPLESS NIGHTS

Just when you think you can enjoy the second trimester and the nausea is a distant memory, the joy of falling into bed can become a military operation.

Firstly there's the constant battle with your mind and body about when you should actually go to bed. We are all guilty of yawning away on the sofa at 9 p.m. but before you know it, it's almost 10.30, you've watched something rubbish on TV, and you have no idea where the time has gone. Then there's the ultimate decision every woman must make before going to bed: to have a hot drink or not. This isn't necessarily about caffeine keeping you awake (but if you're anything like I was, I couldn't even have a cup of green tea before bed without being wide awake for hours) – this is about bladder capacity. Even the smallest amount to drink would send my bladder into overdrive, as just as I was drifting off to sleep an alarm would trigger my overtired brain and scream 'I NEED A WEE!' Cue a huge sigh and loud groan (mainly from my husband) and I would waddle off to the loo, only to find I could wee the same volume as a small hamster. So disappointing. So annoying. On regular occasions.

Babies in the womb have some kind of inbuilt sixth sense that means that as soon you are lying down in a comfortable, relaxed position, it's their cue to throw a party on your bladder. When I was pregnant with the twins I could have sworn they played Twister inside me every night or constantly kicked on my pelvic floor, which would send the most uncomfortable shooting pains on to my cervix.

And as if those things weren't bad enough, there's the battle of the pillows. I didn't actually buy a pregnancy pillow for my last pregnancy as I found previously I got tangled up in it during the night and it made me really hot and sweaty. You may want to try a friend's pillow out before buying one as it may not work for you. But hip and pelvis pain is an unfortunate but common pregnancy ailment. Pregnancy hormones naturally relax your ligaments, the tough tissues that support your joints. And that's because having lax ligaments

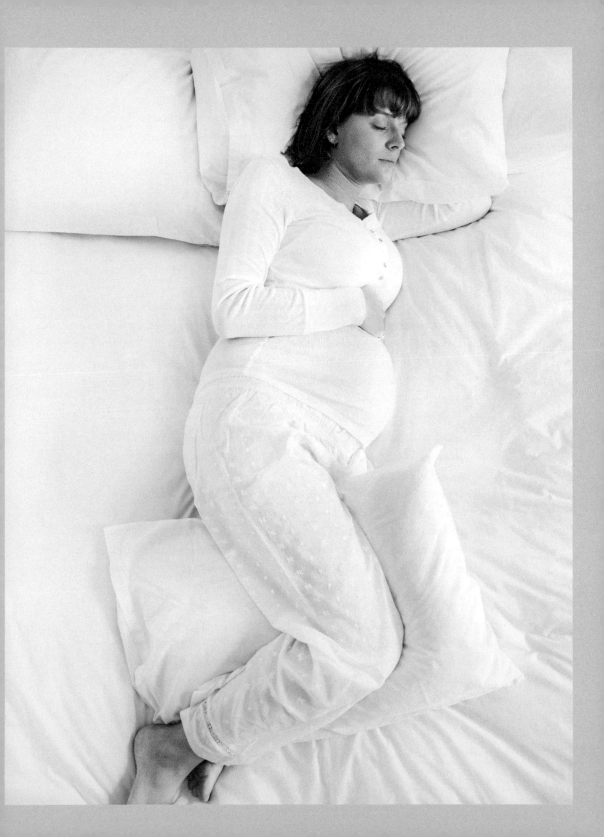

in your pelvis makes it easier for your baby to be born. But this isn't so helpful to hear when it's 1 a.m., you can't get comfy and you have a big meeting first thing in the morning. My first suggestion is to invest in a good mattress. I preferred a firmer mattress, which suited my husband as he has a bad back. The firmer the mattress, the easier it is to turn over in bed, and I also found that my hips didn't sink into the softness of the bed and inevitably start to ache. I then experimented with various spare pillows I already had. Wedging one between my legs was the most comfortable as it kept my hips in line. Other tips for getting a better night's sleep are:

- Start your evening meal earlier. Eating earlier will give you more time for your body to digest your food and therefore you'll be less likely to get heartburn or indigestion. I found eating with my older children at 6 p.m. much better for my digestion – I didn't go to bed feeling sick or as if my pasta was still sitting in my throat.

- Reduce your caffeine intake. Not only do midwives recommend you don't drink more than 200mg of caffeine a day (a cup of tea contains 75mg), but caffeine is a stimulant and the last thing you want to do in the evenings is stimulate your brain more than absolutely necessary. Plus the added liquid volume in your body will only play havoc with your already squished bladder – see above.

- Have a deep, warm bath. I know it's an obvious one but it really can make such a difference. Try adding a few drops of lavender oil to the water, leave your phone downstairs, light some candles and totally zone out of all the stresses you may be feeling. If you can, listen to some hypnobirthing tracks or gentle music through your earphones. The warmth of the water will help ease your aching hips and back, plus you may get some big movements to feel on your bump and it's a lovely way to connect with your baby.

- Switch off your phone, tablet and laptop. We are all guilty of this, but taking those super-useful but super-distracting devices to bed with us means we will inevitably spend at least an extra 30 minutes scrolling through Instagram photos or reading Facebook statuses. Research also shows that blue-light devices can disrupt our natural sleep patterns, so leave your phone in the kitchen or turn on 'flight mode' and pick up a book instead.

HOW YOUR RELATIONSHIP CHANGES

CLEMMIE TELFORD, @CLEMMIE_TELFORD

We all know having a baby affects your body, but few of us can predict quite what it does to your relationship. Here's some of what you can expect:

- Women become mums from the moment that pink line appears on the stick. For partners the 'parental gene' doesn't always kick in straight away. This is irritating, frustrating, maddening and infuriating on so many levels.
- So, even if you've had a modern both-sexes-are-equal-type relationship until now, that will likely go out the window. There's nothing fair about pregnancy and labour. But that's what makes us women the superior sex.
- Seeing your other half talk through your bump to their unborn son/ daughter: 'Hi, Daddy here…' will break your heart.
- A babymoon sounds like a twee idea but, honestly, it is a good one. As is going out on a whim and eating in nice restaurants, as these things don't feel like a big deal now but you will miss them when they have gone.
- Just because you love someone doesn't mean you'll agree on baby names.
- Men tend to like a project. They need help to prepare for labour too: from making sandwiches, to reminding you why you put yourself through it, or stuffing biscuits in your mouth between contractions. Let them help you.
- Not enough of them know about push presents. It may be awful and American and greedy, but a gift in exchange for growing and pushing out a human seems fair, doesn't it?
- He will continue to fancy you in spite of the funny 'ugh' noise you make putting on your shoes, the uncontrolled farting and the crying for no apparent reason during pregnancy.
- And there is a strong chance he will see you poo in labour. But when/if it happens a) you won't care b) he will still love you.
- Being pregnant impacts your relationship in many ways. It changes it and can ruin some bits. But ultimately it binds you together like nothing before.

AM I JUST BUYING FRIENDS?

There are a few key times in your life when meeting and making new friends is a fundamental milestone for building your social circle. It starts on the first day at school: you clock who will be your friend for life based on their hair slides, if they play great imaginary games in the home corner and whether they will invite you to their birthday party. As you get older you start to have a solid group of friends based around who's dating who, which university you went to and where you all live in your early twenties. New jobs bring even more friends and soon you'll find your social circle expanding yet again. So when you become pregnant, you want to meet and know other women who are going through pregnancy at the same time as you, who can share the same experiences and who live close by so you can meet up in coffee shops and swap stories of last night's sleep deprivation.

Antenatal classes are a great way to meet and make these friends, but many come at a cost. The Internet can seem vast and overwhelming, with all the different options available to you. Before you know it, you're not sure if you're merely 'buying friends' or wanting to learn about birth and life with a newborn.

So here are my top tips for choosing the right classes:

- Most of the antenatal groups in the UK are not run by midwives, even the big ones like the National Childbirth Trust. The person who teaches you about how to look after your baby (and yourselves) should have the appropriate training to be able to give you evidence-based information, so always check before booking them.
- All antenatal classes should be open to both you and your partner. This is an opportunity to both learn and the same time meet people going through the same things as you. If a class doesn't accept partners make sure you enquire as to why.
- Recommendations are always great but remember that what was right for

your friend/sister/neighbour may not be right for you and your partner. It can often be 'luck' with who you meet and gel with, so keep options open.

- The NHS offers free antenatal classes either at the local hospital or at your GP's surgery or Children's Centre. These are run by midwives and often include a session just on breastfeeding. They are bigger than private classes and attract people from a larger geographical area, so you may not always meet people who live close to you.

- Consider what you want from classes. If it's just to meet people (perhaps this is your second baby and you've done classes before) then think about other ways in which you can go to meet-ups without paying an expensive fee – maybe use social media to find other mums in your neighbourhood.

- There is a wealth of ways in which you can learn about the process of labour and birth without attending a private course. But make your choices wisely: books are brilliant (as long as they are up to date); speaking to your midwife; and, of course, the Internet is the most obvious and accessible choice. Try to stick to UK-based websites as American ones may not be relevant as to what's on offer here in the UK.

- Keep your eyes peeled in your local café, libraries and cinemas. Noticeboards are a great way to see what's going on in your area. You may find that by doing something like pregnancy yoga or Pilates, you will meet like-minded women who remain your friends once you've had your baby. Local friends are essential when you are desperate to get out of the house and have a coffee and cake with someone, so keep connected!

- Remember that not everyone you meet will become your lifelong friend, so don't go on first impressions. Everyone has different parenting styles and choices, which may not fit with yours, so be open-minded and try not to judge: we're all just figuring this journey in our own way.

28 WEEKS

BYE BYE WAIST

YOUR BABY IS ABOUT THE WEIGHT OF AN AUBERGINE —
JUST OVER 1KG. IT IS AROUND 37.5CM LONG (FROM
HEAD TO TOE, BUT IT IS CURLED UP INSIDE YOU).

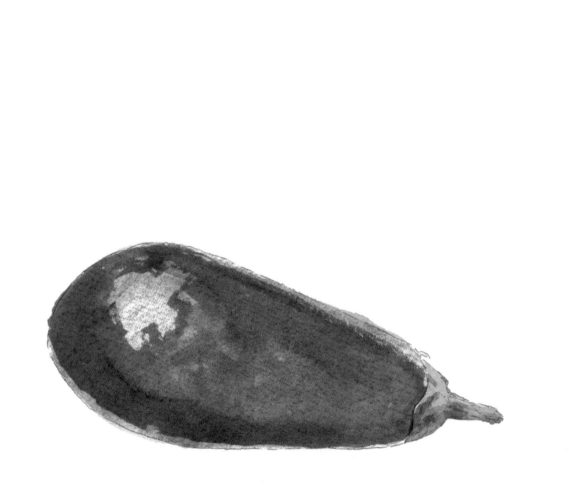

MORE BLOOD TESTS

Just when you thought you were sailing through your pregnancy and enjoying the joys of the second trimester, your midwife offers you another lot of routine blood tests at your 28-week check-up. These blood tests are part of your routine antenatal care and your midwife will explain in detail why you are being offered them. As a quick guide, they include:

- A repeat haemoglobin check (to see how your iron levels are).
- A repeat blood group.
- A random blood sugar; this is to have a look at the glucose levels in your body.

The results of these simple blood tests take a day or two to come back and if there are any concerns your midwife or GP will usually ring you directly. If not, when you see your midwife next they can give you a copy of your result to put in your maternity notes. As with any test you have the right to decline these tests, but make sure you fully understand why your midwife is offering them.

GESTATIONAL DIABETES

Gestational diabetes is a type of diabetes that affects pregnant women, usually during the second or third trimester. It is common and is estimated that 1 in 6 women who give birth in the UK have gestational diabetes. Women with gestational diabetes don't have diabetes before their pregnancy, and after giving birth it usually goes away. The hormones produced during pregnancy can make it difficult for your body to use insulin properly, putting you at increased risk of insulin resistance. And, because pregnancy places a heavy demand on the body, some women are less able to produce enough insulin to overcome this resistance. This makes it difficult to use glucose properly for energy, so the glucose remains in the blood and the levels rise, leading to gestational diabetes. (www.diabetes.org.uk)

Gestational diabetes often doesn't have any symptoms, but you may:
- feel tired
- be very thirsty
- have a dry mouth
- wee a lot
- get recurring infections, such as thrush
- have blurred vision

If you have any of these symptoms, tell your midwife or doctor.

If the random blood test your midwife will offer you at 28 weeks comes back higher than the normal range, they will discuss a further blood test with you. It will be recommended that you have another test called a Glucose Tolerance Test, or GTT, normally carried out at your local hospital. During this test your blood is taken when you haven't eaten anything (usually first thing in the morning); you are then asked to drink a very sugary fizzy drink like Lucozade and a subsequent blood test is taken. The results will determine how your body is coping with high amounts of the sweet stuff and will diagnose whether or not you have gestational diabetes.

Usually the results are given to you on the same day and you'll have a chance to speak to a diabetes nurse, who will go through your diagnosis with you. It may feel very scary and worrying being told you have diabetes, but with good support, healthy eating (one of the biggest changes you can make to your lifestyle is through diet; see pages 16–17), exercise and close monitoring of your blood sugar levels, you and your baby will not be affected.

SWEET TALK

EMMA BARDWELL, HEALTH AND WELLNESS WRITER, @80PERCENTCLEAN

The recommended daily allowance of sugar is six teaspoons (24g), but many of us are consuming at least double that. Sugar isn't just bad in terms of gestational diabetes (see pages 76–7); it also affects your skin, mood, weight, sleep, nails, energy levels and hair. But with the help of a few hacks, you can stop the cravings and break that exhausting cycle of sugar highs and lows. It isn't easy, but the benefits will be felt long after you give birth.

- Cull all sugar-laden products lurking in your cupboards. Look at the labels. There are over 60 names for sugar and most of them end in '-ose'. The most common ones are corn glucose syrup, dextrose syrup and corn syrup.
- Swap milk chocolate for dark; it's mineral-rich, full of antioxidants and contains less sugar.
- It goes without saying that fizzy drinks are a no-no, but so is most shop-bought flavoured water. Make it yourself by infusing water with cucumber, lime, fresh mint, basil or strawberries.
- Eat raw and unprocessed honey, maple/agave syrup, which retain all their natural enzymes. Don't overdo it, as these still contain natural sugars.
- Fruit contains fructose, but because it's bound up in fibre it doesn't cause such drastic blood sugar spikes. Apples, pears and berries are a good bet. Eat with a protein such as nut butter to slow down the release into the blood. Dates are having a moment with health food bloggers, but don't go crazy as they're still very high in natural sugar.
- Cinnamon stabilises blood sugar levels and can help curb cravings. Add it to smoothies and sprinkle it on porridge.
- Smoothies are better than juices as they contain fibre. Try to keep fruit percentages low and veg high.
- Have plenty of healthy snacks in your bag/cupboards/fridge at all times.

I HAD GESTATIONAL DIABETES

BASEER, MUM OF TWO

I was given the diagnosis of gestational diabetes (GD) after a routine 34-week scan. We were devastated, and it was a bit of a horror show at our house for a few weeks as we all went into crisis mode. It was incredibly scary, not helped by the doubling of hospital appointments: our options seemed wiped out and the dream of a natural home birth shattered. I really thought that I had done something to hurt the baby. Because, as mothers, we only hear the worst news, even if it is only a 0.05 per cent risk.

After the initial shock, my natural inclination to fight every battle put things into perspective. There were things I could do and I took every piece of advice going. I was the class geek at the nutritional sessions, scribbling notes. I read every blog on gluten-free food as I figured that I only had six weeks to go, so going without pasta was nothing compared to having a healthy baby.

It was brutal because I am a carb-loving mad pregnant lady. But over time things did become easier. Using equipment to test my blood sugar levels three times a day, I worked out where my levels were and what time of day I could have a piece of fruit without spiking. Few people tell you this, but fruit is literally sugar on a stick. I cut out all carbs, fruit and refined sugar, including diabetic products. Fake sugar is just as bad. And my hard work paid off as I did not need medication. Not being insulin-dependent meant I had options again and I could even negotiate my birth plan.

We no longer have biscuits, chocolate, cake, crisps or even jam in the house. Unless I need it for a recipe I don't buy it. If it's not in the house, we can't eat it. But I don't feel guilty if I do have a big bowl of pasta as a treat. As a family we are all healthier for the diagnosis and I am actually so grateful for the wake-up call.

INCREASING IRON LEVELS

Looking at how your body absorbs iron from the food you consume is a really useful way of knowing how your body is coping with the extra stress of pregnancy. Placentas are very clever at working out what nutrients from food your baby needs to help him or her develop and grow. This, however, may leave your own body with very little iron, even if you eat a ton of red meat and leafy green vegetables. Without enough iron in your blood, the organs and tissues in your body won't get as much oxygen and you may feel really tired and even breathless.

> If you are experiencing tiredness, breathlessness or palpitations always speak to your midwife.

There are several different types of anaemia, but iron-deficiency anaemia is the most common type in pregnancy. About one in seven pregnant women in the UK develop this type of anaemia and you're more likely to develop it if you're carrying twins or more. Your iron levels will have been checked at your booking appointment around 10 weeks into pregnancy. Us midwives like to check that all is hunky dory now so that you and your baby are in good shape for the rest of your pregnancy and birth. If your iron levels are on the low side, don't worry as there are lots of way you can increase them.

DIET

Look again at your diet. Are you really making sure you're eating the right foods and avoiding the wrong foods? Yup, certain foods and drinks can actually make it harder for your body to absorb iron. These include:

- Tea and coffee because of the tannins they contain, so avoid having these with your meals or just afterwards.
- Wholegrain cereals are a good source of iron, but they also contain

phytates that can affect iron absorption, so try to limit these.

- Calcium-rich products, such as milk or yoghurt, also affect iron absorption, so avoid these if you're having an iron-rich meal.

And foods that contain high levels of iron include:

- Red meat, fish and poultry contain iron in a form called haem iron, which your body can easily absorb.
- Foods such as pulses, dried fruit, fortified cereals, wholegrain bread and dark-green leafy vegetables contain iron that is called non-haem iron. This is harder for your body to absorb.
- Vitamin C helps your body to absorb the non-haem iron in food, so drink a glass of orange juice with your cereal. Or combine fruit or vegetables that are rich in vitamin C with ingredients containing non-haem iron.

Sometimes diet alone may not increase your iron levels, and your midwife may recommend that you go to your GP and ask for iron tablets. These are free on prescription. The best time to take them is on an empty stomach, and don't forget the glass of orange juice – it helps your body absorb the iron. Iron tablets do have some unpleasant side effects, which can include:

- Constipation
- Nausea
- Sickness
- Diarrhoea
- Heartburn
- Tummy ache

The tablets may also make your poo darker than usual and even appear black, but try to stick with them and give your body a chance to adjust. Remember that all this preparation now is putting your body in the best possible shape not only for birth but for your post-birth recovery. You don't want any more reasons to feel tired with a newborn baby than necessary.

KICKS COUNT

It's really important to take note of your baby's movements from this stage of your pregnancy until you give birth. You can even download an app to help you keep track of your baby's movements and patterns. The Kicks Count charity have also put together a great guide to ensure you are aware of what's normal and what's not: www.kickscount.org.uk

- There is no set pattern of what is normal as every baby is different, so it is important to get to know your baby's individual pattern. Movements will gradually increase up to 32 weeks, when they will stay the same until birth.

- Babies' movements *do not* slow down as you reach the end of pregnancy.

- During both day and night, your baby has sleep periods that mostly last between 20 and 40 minutes, but no longer than 90 minutes. Your baby will usually not move during these sleep periods.

- There is no set number of kicks that you should be feeling. What is important is that you know what is normal for your baby. There is a common misconception that you should be feeling 10 kicks over a set period, but this is no longer recommended as all babies are different. Babies' movements can vary from 4 to over 100 every hour, so counting to 10 kicks would be irrelevant for most of the population.

- If you notice your baby's movements have slowed down, call your midwife or maternity unit. Do not consume large quantities of something, such as ice-cold water, to prompt your baby to kick as this may lead to indigestion or gurgles you may mistake for movements and give you false reassurance.

- If you are unsure whether or not your baby's movements have slowed down, take some time to focus on them. If you're still unsure, call your midwife or maternity unit. Remember that midwives and doctors will never think you're wasting their time if you notice a change in your baby's movements. Always go and get your baby's heartbeat checked at your local hospital/maternity unit asap and don't wait until the next day.

STYLING YOUR NEW SHAPE

ZOE DE PASS, DRESS LIKE A MUM

At some point you will stop being able to fit into your normal clothes; things will get a bit tighter and a bit uncomfortable – and when you are pregnant it's important to be comfortable both in, and with what, you are wearing. Here are some top tips from pregnancy style blogger, Zoe. www.dresslikeamum.com

- It is worth investing in a few key versatile maternity pieces that can be dressed up and down and worn with what you already have, such as jeans, tights and leggings. If you want to invest in more maternity clothes, make sure that you can breastfeed in them afterwards; you will still be wearing them a few months after the baby arrives, so you want them to last.
- You should already have invested in some decent maternity bras (see page 25) but make sure you reassess the situation as your pregnancy progresses. And buy some nursing bras too.
- Long vests or Lycra dresses are great for wearing under things to help give you more shape and elongate your body. You can even wear your normal T-shirts or tops with a longer vest underneath so that your bump is covered. These are also great for when you are breastfeeding.
- When you're shopping for clothes, think ahead to when the bump has gone. Buy things that you can wear to breastfeed in and post-pregnancy. Shirts are great: if you get them a size or two up you can wear them buttoned up to start with, then towards the end they can be worn open with a top underneath.
- Look through your wardrobe and don't assume you won't be able to fit into any of your clothes, as you might be surprised what fits. Tops that are looser at the bottom are good as you can wear a vest or belly band/ boob tube over your bump and then it won't matter if your top finishes a bit higher up than in your pre-pregnancy days.

- If you are pregnant in the winter invest in a large, warm scarf so that you can wear your normal coats (unbuttoned, when necessary!) and use the scarf to cover your belly. Or consider wearing a cape, where there is plenty of room for a growing bump.
- Get some cool, comfortable trainers – you need to be kind to your feet. From now on they will be carrying more weight, both while you are pregnant and once you are carrying the baby in your arms. Plus, chances are you will be doing a lot more walking and pram-pushing, so you might as well be comfortable and look cool doing it.
- Shoes, bags, jewellery, make-up and accessories are all things you can wear and buy regardless of the size of your bump – embrace them all. Large statement necklaces look great with a pregnant belly, as does a smiling pregnant woman wearing bright-red lipstick.
- Being pregnant and dressing a bump does not mean you have to change your style. There are a lot of things changing inside your body so it is important to feel like yourself on the outside. Do not compromise your style because you are pregnant; stick to what you usually wear but just bump-proof it.
- It is too easy once the baby arrives to forget about yourself, including what you like to wear. Just because you're a mum now, you don't have to dress 'mumsy': you will feel better about yourself if you are feeling confident in what you are wearing.

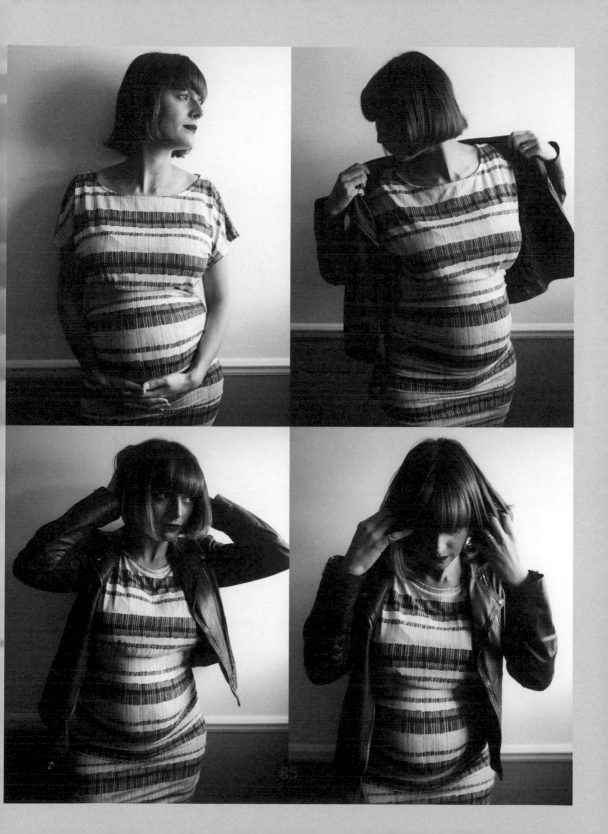

LET'S TALK ABOUT SEX, BABY

There's no subject matter in this book that I'm going to skirt around because it might make you (or me) blush a little, so let's get straight down to business and talk about sex. Sex is such a funny old thing, isn't it? We're still embarrassed of talking about it openly, so much so that when I talk to women post-natally about contraception I don't know who is blushing more, me or the woman. And it's pretty silly, really, as sex is the reason why you're pregnant in the first place. I mean, if it wasn't for sex I would be out of a job and the world would be a very strange place.

During all three of my pregnancies, once the hideous morning sickness had gone, I was up for it. And by 'it' I mean sex. I could have pounced on my husband at any given opportunity. Poor man, he was totally perplexed by the whole matter. In our normal non-pregnant relationship he would have to do a lot of subtle hinting, and like most couples with young children we would have to schedule in the moment when we might be keen; usually if we had a child-free night away or on a mini-holiday. The classic 'I'm too tired' line was often thrown about by either one, or both, of us. But in pregnancy this seemed to be totally irrelevant and I couldn't have been less subtle. Pregnancy hormones made me like a dog on heat. And I'm definitely not alone. Speaking to friends the consensus was that, yes, pregnancy made them all much more horny than ever before!

> I get so horny when I'm pregnant – it's fantastic! This lasts into the third trimester, and only fizzles out when I feel too huge to be physically comfortable. I am able to climax really easily too. Good job, really, as being pregnant also means I'm permanently knackered so it tends to be very short and very sweet, then straight to sleep!
>
> *Louise, mum of two*

I was rampant throughout my pregnancies! I experienced multiple orgasms and we did it a lot more often than when I wasn't pregnant. We even did it twice a day up until I went into labour and I was 10 days overdue.

Sarah, mum of one

It's no surprise that you may find yourself fantasising more about Ryan Gosling, when you consider all those extra hormones swirling around your pregnant body. You have higher levels of the hormones oestrogen and progesterone, which in addition to supporting your continuing pregnancy also increases lubrication in your vagina, blood flow to the pelvic area and the sensitivity of your breasts and nipples; all of which can make you feel like one horny mama.

You may, however, find that your partner might not be as keen to jump into bed. Often men worry about damaging you or the baby (!) during sex. Rest assured, boys, your manhood is never big or long enough to reach where the baby is growing. A simple biology lesson could be useful here – the cervix remains completely closed during pregnancy to prevent the baby from falling out. If, however, your partner is still uneasy about the whole concept, you could stick to foreplay instead. Here are some things to look out for when you're having sex while pregnant:

- You may experience mild contractions during sex and when having an orgasm (or Braxton Hicks), but these contractions are false alarms, and are not powerful enough to start labour, unless it's imminent. These contractions may continue for about half an hour after sex and your uterus will feel rock-hard. They are not dangerous for you or the baby.
- Your uterus may experience spasms during sex, which are different from contractions. This is normal and not harmful.
- You may get cramps during and after an orgasm. Sometimes this is combined with a backache. This, again, is totally normal.

If you experience any fresh bleeding during or after intercourse always speak to your midwife or call your local maternity assessment unit.

31 WEEKS

IT'S ALL ABOUT YOU

YOUR BABY IS ABOUT THE LENGTH OF SOME LONG ASPARAGUS — ABOUT 40CM (FROM HEAD TO TOE, BUT IT IS CURLED UP INSIDE YOU) AND WEIGHS ABOUT 1.5KG.

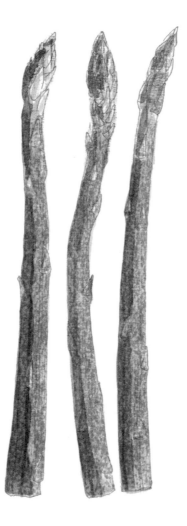

TREAT YOURSELF

This period of time in your pregnancy is what I like to call the 'peaceful time'. Things are ticking on by just fine; you may not have another midwife appointment until 34 weeks but you are most definitely looking pregnant. You should have started your antenatal classes if you decided to go down that route, and met some other expectant parents. It's funny to think that these other women may end up being your lifeline when you're on maternity leave.

That gorgeous bump is growing beautifully and you can still see your ankles, hooray! As I have often said in this book, there is no need to rush around and feel as if you should be doing this or that. Perhaps you've chosen your pram, cot and car seat. Perhaps not: neither is right or wrong, it's just what feels comfortable for you and your partner. I know lots of women who felt too nervous or superstitious buying anything until at least 36 weeks. Remember: THERE ARE NO RULES. Some top tips:

- Invest in some gorgeous lounge wear – you'll be spending more and more time at home resting, so treat yourself and wear something comfortable and soft.
- Book a date night – whether it's going to the local Indian up the road or going away for a long weekend. Most airlines let you fly up until 35 weeks with a singleton pregnancy and 32 with a multiple pregnancy. If you want to go on a flight, remember to get a letter from your midwife or GP.
- Start listening to relaxation tracks. There are lots available online to download – hypnobirthing ones are brilliant, especially just before you go to bed at night, and you and your partner can both listen.
- Talk to your partner. This sounds obvious, but we can spend so much time thinking about baby names, getting the bathroom finished, or buying a new car that actually just sitting down and chatting to them about how they're feeling is really beneficial. When the baby comes along the dynamics will change and your partner may get jealous.

- Take some photos of your bump. Weirdly, you will miss it when it's gone and it's fun to look back over the weeks and see how amazing your body was to carry that baby.
- Moisturise, moisturise, moisturise! And not just your bump: boobs, hips and thighs too. All these areas are changing and expanding and your skin needs all the encouragement it can get. Make this part of your daily skincare routine.
- Treat yourself to a really good pregnancy massage. You will be amazed how good you will feel after having some proper hand action.
- Buy something for your post-pregnancy wardrobe. I invested in my beloved leather jacket. It would take months until it fitted around my boobs but I loved seeing it hanging in my wardrobe and I got a buzz from buying something in a size 10 rather than XXXL. Your body is an amazing thing and it will return to its original shape, or close to it, after you've pushed a human out of it. Amazing.

WHAT IS YOUR PERINEUM AND WHY YOU SHOULD FIND IT!

Yes, perineum. Do you know what it is and where yours is? Sounds like a stupid question, right? But the number of times women (pre- and post-birth) tell me they don't know where theirs is still shocks me!

Most people cringe when they hear the word 'perineum'; it's a bit odd-sounding isn't? Basically your perineum is the piece of muscle and tissue that lies between the bottom part of the vagina and the anus. Prior to having babies, you probably don't ever think about it, but when you're pregnant suddenly your midwife is talking about it like it's public property.

And the reason why midwives talk about it so much is because this is the bit of tissue that has to stretch as your baby's head comes out (crowns). Don't wince! It's amazing how well designed we are as women, however Mother Nature could always do with a helping hand down there. And by help I mean massage. WHAT?! Massage down there during pregnancy? The last area you want to touch or even can physically reach! Yes, I know it sounds all a bit ouchy.

Perineal massage isn't new at all, though: women have been practising it for centuries and research shows it can significantly reduce damage to the tissue during birth. Most women worry about getting stretch marks in pregnancy and the shelves are full of products promising to be the 'magic' lotion or cream to stop them. So why the screwed-up face when I talk to women about massaging down there?

The best time to start perineal massage is around 34 weeks, and I would recommend using an oil such as olive oil, sweet almond oil or sunflower oil.

• Start after you've had a bath or shower as you'll be more relaxed and the tissue will be softer and more comfortable to touch.

- Prop yourself up against some pillows. You can use a mirror if this helps.
- Place your thumbs about 3cm inside your vagina.
- Press your thumbs downward and sideways, gently, until you feel a tingling.
- Hold this stretch for about two minutes.
- Gently massage the lower part of the entrance to your vagina for about three minutes.
- Continue this once or twice a day; after a week you will notice an increase in flexibility and stretchiness.

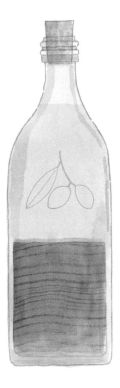

Some people ask their partner to help with perineal massage; my husband looked at me like I was mental and, to be honest, I was quite happy with doing it myself, but if you're both happy to, then go for it! I know some of you reading this may be thinking, 'No way am I going to do this', but seriously it might mean the difference between an intact perineum and needing stitches. So, pregnant ladies, next time you reach for the olive oil when dressing your salad, remember its other uses too.

POSITION OF YOUR BABY

Throughout your pregnancy, your baby will wriggle into all sorts of positions as your uterus grows. By around 35 weeks your baby will begin to sink into the pelvis, ready for birth. Sometimes women say to me that this is around the time they notice a change in their baby's movements. It is usually associated with the change of space around the baby as the head is nicely slotted into the pelvis; those little kicks and punches you used to get change to twists and turns. (But remember, if you notice any change in your baby's movements that causes you concern you should always call your midwife: see page 82.)

The 'occiput anterior' (OA) position is ideal for birth — it means that the baby is lined up so as to fit through your pelvis as easily as possible. The baby is head down, facing your back, with their back on one side of the front of your tummy. In this position, the baby's head is easily 'flexed' i.e. the chin is tucked on to the chest, so that the smallest part of the head will be applied to the cervix first.

The 'occiput posterior' (OP) position is not so good. This means the baby is still head-down, but facing your tummy. Mothers of babies in the 'posterior' position are more likely to have a longer labour as the baby usually has to turn all the way round to face the back in order to be born.

But fear not, because this is the time that you can be doing lots to prevent your baby being in this position for birth. The main culprits are lying back on your soft squishy sofa, sitting in car seats where you are leaning back, or anything where your knees are higher than your pelvis. So the best thing to do this is to spend lots of time kneeling or sitting upright, or on hands and knees. When you sit on a chair, make sure your knees are lower than your pelvis, and your trunk should be tilted slightly forwards.

Here are some ways to help your baby move into the right position:

- Watch TV while kneeling on the floor, over a beanbag/cushions, or sit on a dining chair. Also try sitting on a dining chair facing (leaning on) the back.
- Use yoga positions while resting, reading or watching TV – for example, tailor pose (sitting with your back upright and soles of the feet together, knees out to the sides).
- Sit on a wedge cushion in the car, so that your pelvis is tilted forwards. Keep the seat back upright.
- Don't cross your legs! This reduces the space at the front of the pelvis, and opens it up at the back. For good positioning, the baby needs to have lots of space at the front.
- Don't put your feet up! Lying back with your feet up encourages posterior presentation.
- Sleep on your side (preferably your left) and never on your back.
- Swimming with your belly downwards is said to be very good for positioning babies.
- A birth ball can encourage good positioning of your baby, both before and during labour.

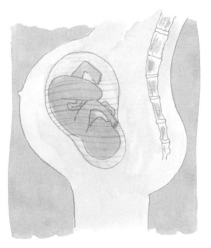

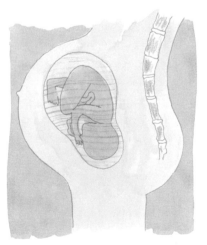

OA   OP

THINKING ABOUT FINISHING WORK

Stopping work can be something to look forward to for some, and something that others may dread. Whatever your take on it, soon enough you simply won't be able to waddle around any longer and your feet and back will be crying out for some respite. You've been lugging your baby around for months and you deserve time off to prepare for the newest member of your family. Here are some signals to look out for that will indicate it's time to hang up the keyboard, take off the uniform and say goodbye to colleagues:

- Commuters on the Tube all jump up and give you a seat due to the size of your bump.
- You spend more time going for a wee than actually writing emails.
- If one more person says 'any day now' in the office you might kill them.
- The elastic in your trousers finally goes and you just don't care.
- You waste time tweaking your labour playlist (see page 145) instead of chasing those all-important invoices.
- You ask yourself: 'Are my maternity trackie bottoms smart enough for work?'
- You wear your maternity trackie bottoms into work the next day and hope your boss doesn't notice.
- You're out of breath by the time you walk down the corridor to the photocopier room.
- Your colleagues find you napping during your lunch break.
- You try to tactically nap behind the screen of your computer.
- You can no longer reach the keyboard on your desk

Hand in your MatB1 certificate to your HR department to get your maternity pay. This is available from your midwife or GP. If you're freelance, find out what you're entitled to on the website below. Don't leave it too late – you don't want to be chasing back payments once your baby is born – you may be a little bit busy. www.gov.uk/maternity-paternity-calculator

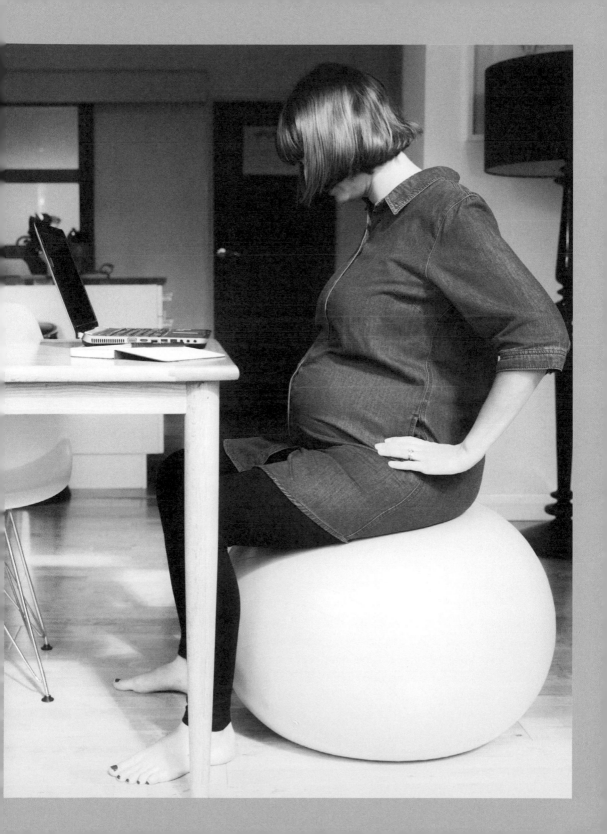

WHAT YOU ACTUALLY NEED TO BUY

These newborn babies only have a few very basic needs: food, sleep and warmth. If you've got those areas covered you will be fine. Collect bits and pieces along the way for when the baby comes so you feel ready, but don't worry if you run out of time: you can buy anything you like online and get next-day delivery – isn't technology wonderful? And you've got your whole maternity leave to go shopping and it's kind of fun buying things for your baby once they have actually arrived. Also you'll be surprised how much you will be given – either new or second-hand – from friends and family.

BABY CLOTHES AND BITS

You don't need much, mainly because you don't really know how big your baby will be – they come in all sizes and scans aren't always reliable.

- 5–10 cotton sleep suits (ideally with closed feet and sewn-in scratch mitts) and 5–10 cotton vests. A combination of newborn and 0–3 months is a good idea in case they turn out to be bigger/smaller than anticipated.
- YOU DON'T NEED SOCKS! They fall off and you'll inevitably lose one and never have a matching pair again, so stick to babygrows with closed feet.
- A few lightweight cotton baby hats – one for when the baby is first born (so prepare for it getting a bit mucky) and one for leaving the hospital in. At home your baby does not need to wear a hat indoors.
- Midwives recommend not using baby wipes on newborn babies as they are heavily scented with chemicals, so go for cotton wool and warm water. Buy a big pack so you can use it for cleaning around baby's face too.
- Nappies. Obviously you need loads, so buy in bulk – better to have more because the moment you put a clean nappy on your baby he or she will, without doubt, poo. EVERY TIME! The alternative is to use reusable nappies; however this does involve a bit more work and, in my experience, the tumble dryer was always on, resulting in bigger energy bills.

- A few cotton cellular blankets (don't buy fleecy ones as they're made of synthetic materials). I'd also recommend buying a few swaddling muslins.
- Muslins are really useful for mopping up sick (theirs) and tears (yours), so buy in bulk — you can never have enough.
- So are dummies. You might be anti them now but withhold judgement until you've experienced extreme sleep deprivation coupled with screamy baby at 4 a.m. Dummies really aren't that bad — in fact they are said to decrease the chance of SIDS. So get a few in, even if only for emergencies.

EQUIPMENT

Again, you don't need to get everything before the baby is born. For example, you don't need to buy a cot until your baby is ready to move into one, which isn't until he or she is around four months old.

- Moses basket or bedside crib — this can be borrowed, but make sure the mattress has a waterproof wipeable cover. And a few fitted cotton sheets.
- A car seat. This is an absolute must, even if you don't own a car. Most hospitals have a policy that you shouldn't leave without your baby in a car seat, even if you're only getting a taxi round the corner. Buy a new one so you can be 100 per cent certain it hasn't been involved in a crash.
- A pram. This is such a personal choice and something many couples disagree about. My husband couldn't believe the price of the pram I tried to convince him to buy first time around (in the end I got it second-hand). If in doubt, go to a large shop that sells all the top brands, test them out and then decide. You will inevitably buy a cheaper, lighter 'stroller'-type buggy when your child turns one, which will be just the job until he or she refuses to go in it. But you don't need this before the baby is born.
- A sling. Check out your local sling library or ask friends if they have one to try. Everyone gets on differently with various styles so try before you buy!
- A changing mat. Ideally one that is plastic-covered and wipe-clean for all those moments (trust me, there will be plenty). If you're pushed for space you really don't need a changing table — a chest of drawers works just fine, or you can easily change your baby on the floor or on your bed.

BOOKING A BABYMOON

SIOBHAN MILLER, @THE_DOUBLE_MAMA

A babymoon is a bit like a honeymoon. Only this time you're at your fattest, rather than your slimmest, and instead of feeling polished and pretty, you've probably not even had a basic wax in months, because, let's be honest, you can no longer see what's going on down there, and you certainly won't remember when you last painted your toenails because that stopped happening around the same time you stopped being able to reach your feet. But saying all that, I still believe it's worth squeezing in a babymoon, whether you're embarking on motherhood for the first or fourth time.

When you have a baby your relationship changes massively (Sherlock, I hear you say) — in fact, all the family dynamics change with a new arrival: an only child becomes a big brother or sister; the baby of the family gets boosted to the unenviable position of middle child; you become a mum of one, or a mum of many. And, of course, with each baby, it becomes even more tricky to find time for the one who used to be your only significant other. So, even if you've got three at home already, however hard it is (logistically, financially, emotionally), it's always going to be easier to find some time to get away before another arrives. So just do it! Find that free weekend, call on Granny, Grandpa, your friend, a neighbour, hopefully-not-a-stranger and get away!

Now, where to go? Somewhere hot, sunny and far-flung? An intrepid adventure? Not so likely. For one, you're probably too pregnant to fly long-haul (check with your doctor or midwife), you're also probably going to want to save that holiday leave for when the baby arrives and you need your other half off work, and then there's the money issue. The long-haul hols might have to be put on a back-burner for a while.

So good ole Blighty! The weather is unpredictable and it may not feel very adventurous, but there are plenty of places that are perfect for your pre-baby getaway. And think of the reduced travel time! 'I love travelling for hours,' said no pregnant woman ever.

Here are my top tips for booking the babymoon of dreams... Ladies, bookmark this page for your partner!

1 FOOD. We know it's essential for every pregnant woman's emotional and psychological well-being but the babymoon is an opportunity to experience culinary delight. There's not a lot left for a heavily pregnant woman to enjoy (sleep, no; sex, probably not by now; all-night raves, no; cocktails, no; skinny jeans, no; sexy lingerie, um...no) but food is still one of them (hurrah!). Find the nicest restaurant you can afford and book it.

2 SPA. A bit of a babymoon cliché, but there's a reason it's such a popular place for pregnant women. When absolutely everything feels heavy and broken and achy, even your vagina, there is literally nothing better than floating like a weightless whale in a warm pool (sans the soundtrack of screaming kids). It's incredible. Leave your inhibitions in the changing room, don that maternity swimsuit and dive in (maybe don't actually dive in). If your spa day includes a treatment, even better. A pregnancy massage is actual real-life bliss (see pages 66–7).

3 Finally, the most important part of your romantic getaway – it's what you dream about day and night while battling insomnia, cramp and reflux, it begins with S... and no, it's not sex, obviously. It's SLEEP! Is there a heavily pregnant woman who wouldn't cut off a limb for a decent night's sleep?! Find a really, really lux hotel to stay in. Even if you can only stay one night and you feel you've blown all your babymoon budget on a bed – do it. Weeks away from giving birth, there is nothing in this world that beats sinking into the most comfortable hotel bed, with more pillows than even a pregnant woman needs, drifting off to sleep dreaming of breakfast served on a silver tray. And if your other half is lucky, he might even get lucky! It's not beyond the realms of possibility that a rested, well-fed, relaxed pregnant woman might be up for it. No guarantees, though.

Check with your midwife or doctor if it's safe for you to fly and that it's safe to have jabs if you need them for your destination. Most airlines require a letter confirming this. And don't forget your maternity notes!

WHY HYPNOBIRTHING IS THE BEST TOOL FOR LABOUR AND BIRTH

HOLLIE DE CRUZ, LONDON HYPNOBIRTHING AND @THEYESMUMMUM

Although a lot of people are put off by the slightly bats name, 'hypnobirthing' is, in fact, the most logical, gentle and profound form of birth education I have come across. At its core, hypnobirthing combines an education in the physiology and the psychology of birth. You will learn exactly how your birthing muscles are designed to work during labour, how your hormonal responses affect them, and how to put yourself back in control of the two.

Mammals are designed to give birth comfortably and efficiently. Sadly though, in Western culture we are bombarded from an early age with images that portray birth as traumatic and painful. Our subconscious mind stores these messages and when we become pregnant and go into labour, a fight-or-flight mechanism is triggered to protect us from the perceived danger ahead. The production of adrenalin diverts blood and oxygen to our defence systems, and away from our reproductive system, meaning our birthing muscles become deprived of the fuel they need. These muscles become tired and tense, creating painful contractions that confirm our initial fear of how awful birth is. If we can short-circuit this adrenalin production, our birthing muscles will get what they need to work harmoniously.

With that in mind, a big part of hypnobirthing is about giving your subconscious mind a bit of a clear-out. You will explore where your fears of birth come from and release unhelpful beliefs. You will then begin to reprogramme your subconscious by looking at how other mammals and women in other parts of the world birth with more ease; by using daily positive affirmations; and surrounding yourself with healthy imagery of birth.

Birth partners can all too often feel like a bit of a spare part and hypnobirthing changes that too. You will both learn simple but specific deep relaxation, massage and breathing techniques. You will learn how to communicate with caregivers, make informed decisions and put yourselves back in control of your birth. You will be equipped to navigate the turns of your labour in a way that means you feel confident, calm and empowered. Involving the birth partner in this way not only makes for a more enjoyable pregnancy together, but also means that when you go into labour, you will feel fully supported so that you really can tune in to what your body wants from you, even if you're someone who naturally finds it difficult to switch off.

Hypnobirthing doesn't promise a perfect birth, but it will give you the best birth for you and your baby at the time, and if you commit to even small amounts of daily practice, you will create a positive, joyful experience that will stay with you and your baby for the rest of your lives.

Hypnobirthing, for me, is not about 'should'; it's about empowerment. While courses are generally geared towards natural births with minimal interventions, what is taught are tools, not ideals. And part of natural birth is the unexpected twists and turns it can sometimes take. It's all about teaching women to trust their instincts, ask questions, make informed decisions and follow the lead of their bodies. To trust their birth partner, to work in harmony with their baby, to create the best birth environment possible. So if you're pregnant and reading this, please don't just wing it. Equip yourself with a big toolbox of knowledge and techniques to give you confidence and self-belief to use throughout pregnancy, birth and beyond into motherhood. Your baby's birth stays with you for ever: for it to be powerful and positive is life-changing.

One easy exercise to do at home is a breathing technique called 'up-breathing'. You can use this during your pregnancy to help calm the mind and relax the body, and also during the early stages of labour (see pages 122–3). Close your eyes, relax your body, inhale through your nose to a count of four and then out through your nose to a count of six. A longer exhale will immediately work to quieten your mind and shut out distractions, helping you to maintain focus and calm. Be sure to breathe into your stomach, rather than chest. Your shoulders should remain soft and relaxed.

34 WEEKS

FEELING CONFIDENT, FEELING PREPARED

YOUR BABY WEIGHS ABOUT THE SAME AS A PINEAPPLE — 1.9KG. IT IS AROUND 43.5CM LONG (FROM HEAD TO TOE, BUT IT IS CURLED UP INSIDE YOU).

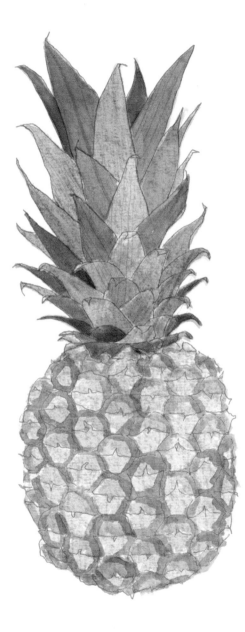

YOUR GROWING AND CHANGING BODY

You've made it to 34 weeks! You may feel like you've been pregnant for ever but the big day is less than two months away. It can sometimes feel a bit like your body is changing out of your control, which you may be finding difficult to cope with. Try to remember that any weight you gain in pregnancy is for your baby and can easily be lost via breastfeeding and exercise. You'll be amazed how much pram-walking you'll do with a new baby, so now's a good time to invest in some comfortable trainers; I got to know my local area very well after my babies were born! (Although do also remember that you only really need an extra 200 calories per day in the third trimester.)

You may notice the extra weight you gain is focused around your back, abdomen and upper thighs (the places us women are always trying to shift it from). These fat stores provide a reserve of calories for you and your baby to use in the last six weeks of pregnancy. They will also be used when you are breastfeeding. I know this doesn't make it any easier when your usual slender frame looks a little different in the mirror, but try to focus on why these changes are happening and embrace your beautiful new shape. Your partner will no doubt be in awe of what an amazing job you are doing – and so should you be!

Other changes to your body may include:

• Your belly button may change from an 'innie' to an 'outie'.
• You may start to leak a few drops of colostrum onto your bra or pyjamas – this is a sign that your breasts are starting to produce milk.

By around 34 weeks your baby weighs around 4lbs, but you probably feel as if you weigh around 400lbs! You may have noticed your bladder has become your baby's trampoline and frequent trips to the loo day and night have become a normal part of your life (despite you only ever being able to produce a measly amount of wee each time). Your midwife will measure your bump at every antenatal check with a tape measure – from your pubic bone to the top of your uterus – to see how things are growing. On average, your uterus should grow 1cm a week and match the number of weeks' pregnant you are, but it's still within normal limits if you measure 2cm above or below this. If your midwife is worried about how much you are measuring she may refer you for a growth scan at the hospital, just to be on the safe side. Some hospitals routinely offer a third scan between 34 and 36 weeks; this will depend on the area you're living in.

Your baby's movements may change around now. If your baby is 'head down' it may feel a little more uncomfortable in your pelvis, especially when walking for long periods of time. If your baby is breech (bottom first) you may get a strange sensation of a hard head under your ribcage. Try not to worry too much if your baby is in the breech position at this stage; your midwife will discuss with you your options at your next appointment (see page 156). However, your baby should continue to move normally throughout your pregnancy and you should even continue to feel the movements while you are in labour, although you'll be focusing on breathing during those contractions. As they get bigger, the movements feel different but they should still follow their usual pattern right up to the end. It is not true that babies 'slow down' as labour approaches, but they do have less space to move in. Remember to report any change of movements to your midwife immediately (also see page 82).

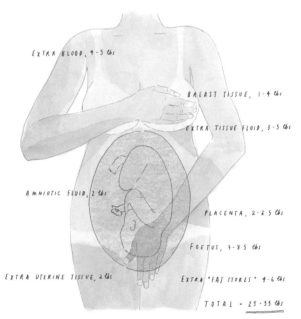

EXTRA BLOOD, 4-5 lbs

BREAST TISSUE, 1-4 lbs

EXTRA TISSUE FLUID, 3-5 lbs

AMNIOTIC FLUID, 2 lbs

PLACENTA, 2-2.5 lbs

FOETUS, 7-8.5 lbs

EXTRA UTERINE TISSUE, 2 lbs

EXTRA "FAT STORES" 4-6 lbs

TOTAL = 25-35 lbs

INFANT FEEDING

It's never too early to start thinking about how you are going to feed your baby. The feeding choices you make will be personal to you and your circumstances. It takes time to adjust to your new role as a parent and what works for one mum and baby may not necessarily work for you. And you know what? That is okay. Every mum's experience of feeding their baby will be different, just as every baby is different. Understanding and educating yourself will help you make the right choices later on when your baby is actually here.

BREASTFEEDING

Breastfeeding has many benefits, and babies who breastfeed are at a lower risk of:

- Gastroenteritis
- Respiratory infections
- Sudden infant death syndrome (SIDS)
- Obesity
- Type 1 & 2 diabetes
- Allergies (e.g. asthma, lactose intolerance)

And for mothers the benefits include protection against:

- Breast and ovarian cancer
- Hip fractures in later life
- Heart disease
- Obesity

Breastfeeding is a skill and education and empowerment are key. Take the pressure off yourself and give yourself space, time and kindness. Prioritise getting to know your baby away from situations that make you question your ability. And always ask for help – there is plenty of support out there.

FORMULA-FEEDING

You may already know that you want to formula-feed your baby and just like breastfeeding, you should be supported in your decision by those around you. Make sure you understand how to correctly formula-feed. These include:

- The correct way to sterilise and make up the feeds
- Which type of bottle and formula milk to buy
- How much you should be feeding your baby
- Understanding responsive feeding as opposed to scheduled
- Following your baby's hunger cues

Some women may feel worried that they won't bond in the same way if they formula-feed, but there are many ways to still enjoy the closeness between you and your baby when formula-feeding, which can include skin-to-skin feeding and close cradle-holding, where you place the baby's head in the crook of your arm and your other arm around the baby or underneath them.

Remember that the most important thing is that a baby is fed safely. Whether that's exclusive breastfeeding, mixed feeding or formula, how you feed your baby is an individual's choice and not for others to judge. There is no one-size-fits-all solution and often it can seem like a case of trial and error. There's a wealth of information and support out there, whether you decide to breastfeed or formula-feed your baby.

POSITIVE BREASTFEEDING

IMOGEN UNGER, LACTATION CONSULTANT AND SENIOR NEONATAL INTENSIVE CARE NURSE

It's amazing that already your body is making milk that will nourish your baby after he or she is born. You have everything you need to breastfeed your baby. Below are some tips to help you prepare for a positive experience.

- Finding out the basics of breastfeeding is a great place to start. Find out how your body makes milk and the many different ways you can hold your baby to breastfeed.

- Understand what newborn feeding behaviour looks like. Issues and concerns seem to arise when things are perceived as being a problem, when in fact they are just normal newborn behaviours. Knowing that these things, for example frequent feeding, cluster feeding and growth spurts, are part of normal newborn development will give you confidence to make the best decisions for your baby.

- Familiarise yourself with what feeding cues look like so you can recognise when your baby is hungry. Understanding what their stomach size is at different ages will help make sense of your baby's frequent feeding.

- There are some great resources, including online videos of babies breastfeeding. These can provide accessible support and guidance. Make a list of these now, plus other websites, the contact numbers of helplines and locations of local support groups. Hopefully everything will go really well and you won't need them, but if you do need added support because breastfeeding is taking a while to get going, you will know where to turn.

- Know that, with the right support, most mothers can make enough breast milk for their baby. The information you discover now, from the right sources, will inform and empower you when making feeding choices for your baby.

- Be confident and trust that your body, which nurtured your baby for the duration of this pregnancy, can continue to do so once he or she is born.

WHAT YOU REALLY NEED

The shops are full of breastfeeding paraphernalia, which leaves women asking: 'Do I really need an all-singing all-dancing double-electric breast pump before the baby is even earthside?' A bit of boob investigation at this stage wouldn't go amiss. Have a good look at your boobs. Do your nipples point outwards or are they flat or even inverted? Have you had breast surgery, which may affect where the milk is produced? Chat things through with your midwife, as it is good to be prepared for any obstacles that may be thrown your way during your breastfeeding journey. Here's a list of things you definitely need and things you can hold off buying, or not buy at all.

- A really decent feeding bra, or two: ideally one to wear in the day and one to wear at night. The better quality, the longer it will last. It's amazing how many times you'll clip and unclip that little plastic device.
- Breast pads. In the beginning, when your boobs are still adjusting to all the feeding, they will spontaneously leak, so stock up on a load of pads.
- Good-quality lanolin-based nipple cream. Chances are your nipples haven't endured the constant wear and tear feeding a newborn baby can cause. It's a bit like a new pair of shoes – they can rub and blister at first and then wear in and are the most comfortable shoes you've ever worn.
- A breastfeeding pillow. This is one thing I'd say you don't necessarily need. I borrowed one with my first baby and didn't get on with it, so with my second I made do with the cushions I had lying around the house.
- A breast pump and bottles. See how breastfeeding goes before buying these. There are electric and manual breast pumps available and not everyone gets on with a certain type. As long as it's sterilised you can also buy second-hand or hire a breast pump from a local source.
- A steriliser. These are big and cumbersome and take up a lot of space. You can easily use boiling water in a saucepan to sterilise bottles as a short-term solution before deciding if you really need to buy one.

AND WHAT'S THE ALTERNATIVE?

No one can really predict how feeding your baby is going to go; it's a skill both you and your baby need to learn. Sometimes, for whatever reason, there are obstacles that may make it harder for you to breastfeed and you may decide that breastfeeding isn't the right thing for you or your baby. You may know already that you're planning on bottle-feeding from the word go. Or you may end up using a combination of breast milk and formula. Whichever way you decide to feed your baby make sure you're 100 per cent supported by those around you. Being a new mum is hard, so be kind to yourself.

GABRIELLA, MUM OF ONE

I really struggled in the early days of breastfeeding. My daughter Etty was a 9lb 1oz hungry, screaming, feeding machine and my dwindling milk supply was met with angry fists and tears all round. For three weeks we battled through, armed with tubes of lanolin, attending breastfeeding support groups, watching Internet videos on the perfect feed position, thanking the Lord for gel nursing pads, and subjecting my poor daughter to a snip when it emerged that she had a tongue-tie and was therefore hindering our journey to breastfeeding bliss.

In the end I simply reached for the formula. After many sleep-deprived sessions, I decided that it was healthier to rein in the stress, fill my daughter's tummy and focus less on what wasn't happening for us and more on enjoying the early days with my newborn. I combine-fed until Etty was about four months old, and formula-fed exclusively from then on. If and when baby number two comes along of course I'll attempt to breastfeed, but I'll be much less scared of reaching for the formula if needs be. Happy mama, happy baby and all that…

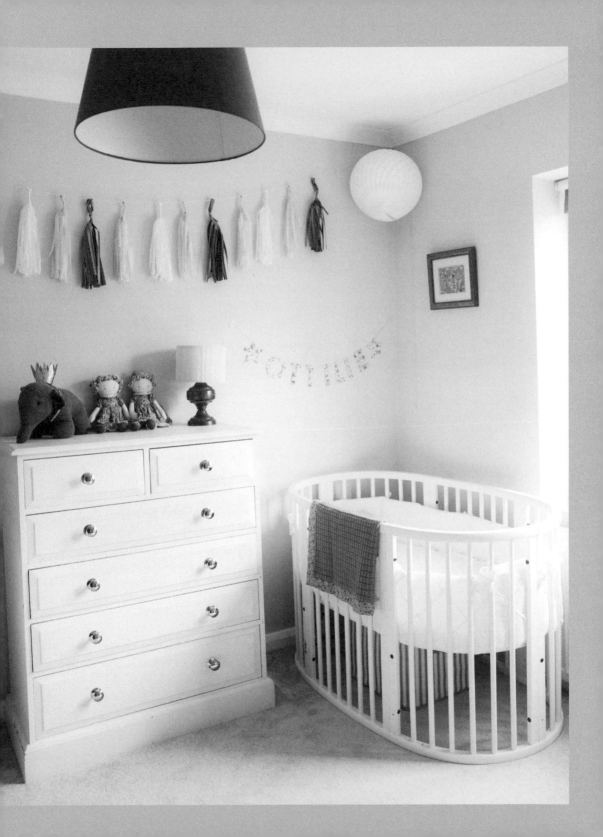

PRE-ECLAMPSIA

Pre-eclampsia is a rare but serious condition that affects around 6 per cent of women during their pregnancy. It causes high blood pressure and it also causes protein to leak from your kidneys into your urine. When you see your midwife for your antenatal appointments they will routinely check your blood pressure and dip your urine with a stick to check for the presence of protein.

You may have no symptoms at first, or you might have only mildly raised blood pressure and a small amount of protein in your urine. If pre-eclampsia becomes worse, one or more of the following symptoms may develop. Contact your midwife urgently if any of these occur:

- Severe headaches that do not go away.
- Problems with your vision, such as blurred vision, flashing lights or spots in front of your eyes.
- Abdominal pain. The pain that occurs with pre-eclampsia tends to be mainly in the upper part of your abdomen, just below your ribs, especially on your right side.
- Vomiting later in your pregnancy (not the morning sickness of early pregnancy).
- Sudden swelling or puffiness of your hands, face or feet.
- Not being able to feel your baby move as much.
- Just not feeling right.

MOLLY GUNN, @SELFISHMOTHER
At the end of 2010, my first pregnancy was happening in textbook fashion and I was in a glow of excitement. We had done a hypnobirthing course in preparation for a home birth, and with a few months until our 22 March due date, I spent lots of time researching

birth pools and composing a soundtrack. But, a few days later, a case-loading midwife came to my house, took one look at my swelling ankles and told me about this thing I'd never heard of: pre-eclampsia. She said that if you have swollen ankles, protein in your urine and high blood pressure, it is bad. She told me to call her if I started to feel 'different'. Nope, I thought, I'm absolutely fine, and I carried on as usual. Except... soon I did start to feel different. My face started swelling, and I could only wear flip-flops because my feet were so big. My head ached and I felt really, really heavy. A week after her visit I called her. It was Valentine's Day.

'I don't feel right,' I said.

'Get to the hospital now,' she said.

'But, the food delivery is coming,' I said, 'I've ordered scallops!'

At the hospital the midwife laughed when I said I was cooking scallops that night. She also laughed when I said I was having a home birth. 'You're not going anywhere,' she said, as she put me in a bed on the labour ward.

Every day I pretended I wasn't really ill. Yet, my blood pressure and protein count kept getting higher. Then I started swelling beyond recognition. My entire face and body puffed up so much I could hardly see out of my puffy eyes. A friend from NCT came in to have her baby and didn't recognise me. I asked every day to go home but the midwives shook their heads. 'I'll be fine!' I insisted. But one morning, I admitted defeat: I felt dizzy, my eyesight went blurry and my head was pounding. I had reached 36 weeks, so the midwives induced me, otherwise my organs would start shutting down. Things happened slowly before I was epiduraled to the eyeballs and spent 12 (very chilled) hours in a labour room, with Fleetwood Mac, and Tom massaging my feet. But, when Rafferty's heart rate went funny they whizzed us into the operating theatre and whipped him out. He was 5lb and gorgeously healthy.

RELAXATION TECHNIQUES

In your busy life you probably find it difficult to put aside the time to relax. We don't tend to switch off the way that we should. But by this stage of your pregnancy it's a really good idea to start making time to relax, whether it's taking a glorious hot bath at the end of a long week or going to bed early with your favourite book – because just taking a few minutes out of your day, away from your phone and laptop, is really beneficial for you and your pregnancy.

Whether this is your first or fourth baby, it's never too late to find space in your day. A few good ways of relaxing include:

- Swimming – many women during pregnancy find going for a gentle swim a lovely way to switch off (you can't take your phone into the pool with you) and the water creates support for your bump, so you feel weightless.
- Massage – I honestly think pregnancy massage should be offered free on the NHS for all women. I had these regularly through my pregnancy and I came away each time feeling soft and floaty and was guaranteed a good night's sleep too. Win–win. My husband also learnt some basic massages from watching videos online, so you can do this on the cheap as well. You just need someone who is willing and able. (Also see page 67.)
- Fresh air – a great motto I use as a mother is 'If in doubt, go out' and this is true for pregnancy too. If your house is a mess and driving you mad, or you can't manage to get those chores done, go for a walk. Not only will the exercise do you good, getting fresh air into your lungs and vitamin D on your face is good for the soul. You may not be able to be as spontaneous once the baby arrives, so make use of this free time while you can.
- Meditation, whether this is guided in your yoga class or in private when listening to a download, can really help you to let go of any worries and anxiety you may be having. Pregnancy creates a rollercoaster of emotions fuelled in part by raging hormones, which make you feel excited one

minute (yay! a tiny human is going to arrive at the end of this) to completely terrified the next (OMG, will my life ever be the same again?). It is super-helpful to relax your body, mind and soul and is the perfect exercise to do during pregnancy. It also allows you to take the time to connect with your bump and baby, something that during your busy day you may have not had time to do.

We breathe in and breathe out every single moment without realising its importance. It's subconscious but hugely beneficial, and that's why meditation can help focus on our breathing, relax muscle tension and reduce stress. These skills will come in useful when you're in labour, so now is a great time to start practising.

Here are some tips for getting into meditation practice:

- Turn off your phone and any other noises that may distract you.
- Sit down in a comfortable position with your eyes closed.
- Gently place your hands on your bump from beneath and breathe deeply. Feel your bump rising each time you breathe.
- You will also feel the movement inside yourself. Breathe through your nose and close your mouth.

Alternatively, you can do this exercise when you're lying in bed or even when you're submerged in a deep, warm bath. It really doesn't matter where you choose to practise, as long as you feel calm and relaxed. 'Inhale peace, exhale tension' is a great sentence to repeat while using this simple breathing technique.

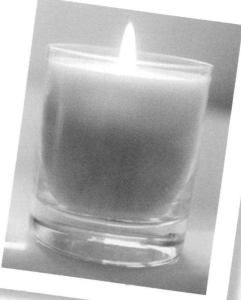

36 WEEKS

IS THERE REALLY GOING TO BE A HUMAN AT THE END OF THIS?!

YOUR BABY IS ABOUT THE SIZE OF A ROMAINE LETTUCE — 47.5CM (FROM HEAD TO TOE, BUT IT IS CURLED UP INSIDE YOU) — AND WEIGHS MORE THAN 2.5KG.

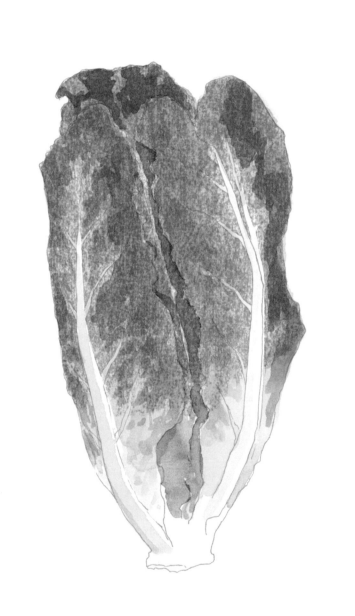

WRITING YOUR BIRTH PLAN

I don't like the word 'plan'. Any plans you make in life – weddings, job interviews, holidays – almost never go exactly the way you thought they would. You have to expect the unexpected. So rather than 'planning', think of it more as 'preparing'. This is why I use the term 'birth preferences'. A birth preference is a much more positive way of looking at labour and birth. We'd all prefer sunny skies on our wedding day but you can't let rain ruin the day.

The aim of a birth plan is to communicate your wishes to the people who will care for you in labour. It's a nice way for us midwives to get an idea of what a couple is like, especially if we haven't met them before. We're pretty good at getting to know couples fairly quickly in a short space of time! There are no hard-and-fast rules for how to do it, but below are some good starting points. Remember, though, that births can be unpredictable, and if you've not experienced it before, then you may well feel differently on the day. So allow for flexibility. The best way of ensuring things go to plan is by acknowledging that they may not always go to plan.
• Do your research: find out what's likely and what's possible where you have chosen to give birth (see chapter 3).
• Gather information but fight the fear: understand the process and reality of birth but don't get bogged down in labour stories from hell. This is your baby's birth! Fear is your enemy; kick it to the kerb now.
• Talk to your birth partner: explore what both your priorities are, and if there's anything you're worrying about, address it together.

Discuss and write your birth plan with your birth partner, so you are on board together. For example, you need them to know and understand why you may not want to be lying on your back for the pushing stage, or why pethidine isn't a great option if you're hoping to stay active and use the pool. During labour you want someone to be your advocate and voice. Labour is hard work and requires all your energy and focus. You don't want to have to answer the midwife's questions mid-contraction. And always allow for a change in your preferences, i.e. 'I'd like to use the pool for labour but if it is recommended that I need to be continuously monitored I would like to stand/use the ball/ use the mat/sit on a chair so I'm not on the bed.' Keep your options open. Now jot some things down – some key things to consider:

- Who is your birth partner? Where do you want them to be, when?
- What positions do you want to consider for labour/birth? (see pages 46–7)
- Pain relief and what order you'd like it in: include here any specifics like hypnobirthing techniques or massage (see pages 102–3 and 201).
- What you want to do in the event that labour has slowed?
- Do you want to use a pool or any other equipment, e.g. birthing ball?
- Do you want baby monitoring? If so how are you happy for this to happen?
- Do you want a Managed or Natural Third Stage (placenta delivery)? See: www.nice.org.uk/guidance/cg190/ifp/chapter/delivering-the-placenta
- Who do you want to cut the cord?
- Do you want skin-to-skin when the baby is born, if possible?
- Vitamin K for your baby – oral drops or injection? (Talk to your midwife.)
- What are your hopes and requests for feeding your baby?
- What do you want to happen in unexpected situations? For example, if your baby needs to go to SCBU do you want your birth partner to go with them or stay with you?
- Any particular requirements, e.g. religious needs or language difficulties?

Pop a copy of your birth preferences in your maternity notes and make sure your partner shows it to your midwife when you're in labour. As the big day approaches, go back and review your choices to make sure it's still what you want. Remember, you can always change your mind. And don't put too much pressure on yourself: if you need an epidural because you've been in early labour a long time and had no sleep, then that's what's right for you at that point. Never feel guilty or beat yourself up about the choices you've made, because they will always be the right choice at the time.

STAGES OF LABOUR

LABOUR IS EXACTLY LIKE A MARATHON,
THE HARDEST MARATHON YOU'LL EVER RUN

I think it's really important to know and understand the stages of labour, what will happen and when key things will happen. This will help you to know when to go into hospital/phone for a taxi/call the community midwives (if you're planning a home birth). But like anything, biology doesn't always follow the rules and if this isn't your first baby, times and lengths of labour may differ. Remember that we are all made up differently and don't perform in exactly the same way.

First stage or early/latent phase
This is usually the longest stage of labour so it's probably the stage that you should understand the most. However it's usually the stage that the majority of first-time mums overlook. I always like to tell women that labour is like running a marathon (I've never run a marathon myself but I have gone through three, well, four labours if you count both of the twins). You never start a marathon using up all your resources and energy; you start slowly, pacing yourself as best you can. Labour is no different.

So let's start with a carrot, because your cervix is like a small carrot. It's not orange but it's long and firm, and by the time you're in established or active labour (5cm dilated) it's completely changed shape. It's moved forward, shortened, opened, dilated and softened. Imagine your cervix is now like the opening of a sock. So that's quite a bit of change it's got to make and this is why it can take several days of early labour to do so. During the first stage of labour you may experience:
• Backache, period-type pains.
• A vaginal bloody show (the mucus plug that sits in the neck/opening of the cervix).

- Short irregular contractions.
- Your waters might break (but these can break at any stage of labour, even as the baby is being born).
- Diarrhoea, nausea or you may even actually vomit.

A contraction can feel like a stronger version of a period pain, but everyone feels them differently.

> It felt like griping pains, like when you have a bad stomach bug. It came and went and built in intensity and my tummy went really hard, like a big rock!
>
> *Louise, mum of one*

Women often get really excited when they think they're going into labour, and why not? Of course it's exciting – but remember the marathon analogy: **take it slowly**. If your contractions are short and far apart you are not going to push a baby out any time soon.

Watch your UFO

When thinking of the best positions for labour, remember UFO: U for Upright, F for Forward and O for Open. Any position where you are upright, forward and open is great. When upright you obviously have gravity on your side, and by leaning forward you're encouraging the baby into the optimum position for birth, as the weight of the back of the baby's head will be round to the front of you as opposed to resting against your back. By open I mean your legs are apart and you are creating room in your pelvis rather than restricting the space. This will make life, or at least labour, easier for you.

Some really useful things to do to help you through this stage include:

- SLEEP/REST: The number of women I know who charge around the park or walk up and down the stairs from the first twinge baffles me. Doing that, you will without doubt completely exhaust yourself. If it's early labour, rest while you can. If the contractions slow down and stop altogether go to bed or make a nest on the sofa, draw the curtains, switch off your phone, and smell some lavender. You will be so grateful for any snippets of sleep you can grab now and your body will thank you for it when it really needs the energy later on.
- DISTRACTION: If your partner is at home with you, stick on your favourite box set. Why not stand and do some cooking? (Remember UFO – Up, Forward, Open.) This will help the baby to get into a good position in your pelvis. Plus a home-made lasagne in the fridge will be very much welcomed when you come home from hospital and are starving hungry!
- EAT/DRINK: When you're in established labour, you're less likely to feel hungry, so eating and staying hydrated in early labour is vital. You need food that is jam-packed with slow-releasing energy: porridge with fruit and honey, a big bowl of pasta, and peanut butter on toast are great. Coconut water is full of antioxidants and great for when you need hydrating. (Make sure you pack some in your hospital bag, see pages 52–3.)
- RELAX: Get in the deepest bath possible, light a candle, put on your hypnobirthing tracks and stick a pair of headphones in your ears. Switch off from the world and focus on your baby and body. It's doing an amazing thing but it takes time, so don't try to rush it. Practising your breathing exercises at this stage is a fantastic way to find your rhythm so that you find it much easier to use later on, when labour is established.
- MASSAGE: Now is the perfect time to get your partner to show off their massage techniques. Remember to focus on your shoulders, lower back and feet. (See pregnancy massage, page 67.)

You may begin to notice a rhythm or pattern with the contractions, so you could start to time them using an online app or just getting your partner to jot them down. As a rough guide, contractions in early labour are usually more than 5 minutes apart and only last between 20 and 30 seconds. Remember, if they are short and irregular it's probably too soon to be thinking about calling your midwife or going to the hospital. You'll only be disappointed if you go in too soon and are sent home again.

So when should you to go to the hospital/call your midwife if you're planning a home birth?

- First baby: your contractions are every 3 minutes, lasting at least 40 seconds and are **strong** and **regular**.
- Second baby: your contractions are every 5–7 minutes but are **strong** and **regular**.

Remember you should always call your midwife if:

- You have a heavy 'show' of bright-red blood (heavier than a period).
- You feel your waters breaking (this is when the amniotic fluid leaks out through your vagina), especially if they are brown, green or smelly.
- Your baby's movements slow down.
- You are worried about anything.

Active phase

This is when you're in business and hopefully labour won't stall or stop if you've remained as rested as possible in the early/latent phase. You may already be in the hospital at this point, or your midwife will have come to your home if you're planning a home birth. You will be offered a vaginal examination to assess how dilated (open) your cervix is at this point. Try not to focus too much on this, though: it's just a number and doesn't necessarily determine how long your labour will be. Remember, your body is amazing and your cervix is now dilated at least 5cm. Your contractions are strong and regular, coming about every 3–4 minutes and lasting at least 45 seconds. You may feel these contractions in your back or across your uterus and won't be able to talk through them; up-breathing (see hypnobirthing, pages 102–3) is brilliant for getting through these contractions. It's important to remain (if possible) upright for this stage, rather than lying on your back, as you want your baby's head to be well applied to your cervix to encourage dilation.

If you have had an epidural by this point, ask your midwife and partner to encourage you to change position on the bed; lying on your left side and even going on your knees and leaning over the back of the bed is really beneficial. If you're mobile (which may not be the case if you've had an epidural) ask to use a birthing ball, mats and bean bags – in hospital they may not be visible but are often kept in storage cupboards.

As the contractions are now closer together a few useful tips on how to manage the gaps in between include:
• Small sips of water or coconut water via a sports bottle or cup with a straw.
• Try to empty your bladder every hour as a full bladder can make it harder for your baby to get into a good position (sitting on the loo is a good position to try for a bit).
• Keep lighting low and noises minimal – you want to feel safe and calm.
• Wiggle your hips and pelvis to keep everything loose and open.
• If you're in the pool ask your partner to pour warm water over your neck and shoulders.

Contractions in the active phase tend to maintain their momentum and open your cervix more rapidly, but it may still be many hours before your cervix is fully dilated. Take it one step at a time and remember that each contraction is bringing you closer to meeting your baby. You can do it!

Transitional phase

This is when you move from the first stage of labour to the second stage. It usually starts when your cervix is about 8cm dilated, and ends when your cervix is fully dilated, or when you get the urge to push. Your contractions may space out a bit but are much stronger and longer-lasting. It's common for waters to break just before, or during, transition. As your cervix becomes fully dilated, you may have another show of blood.

As women experience transition in different ways it's hard to tell how you will be. Try to remember that it's okay to feel scared, vulnerable, overwhelmed and emotional. You may feel zoned in to your labour and only able to make abrupt demands (I snapped at my husband many times at this stage). You may make noises that you can't control, you may shout and feel impatient with everyone, but this is okay: your body is about to do something amazing. Your midwife will be very experienced at knowing how to support you and your partner during this stage.

If you're planning to give birth without pain relief, this may be the most testing part of labour for you and your birth partner. You may want to tear up your birth plan or demand an epidural, even though you'd hoped to avoid one! Or if you'd planned a home birth, you may now want to go to hospital. All of these feelings are normal and with lots of support and encouragement from your midwife and partner you will get through this next stage – your baby will be born soon!

> During my home birth I asked for someone to get my shoes and coat as I wanted to go to hospital. I have no idea why I wanted to go; it was just something I kept saying. Obviously there was no clinical reason why I should be transferred and before I could think about anything else, the sensation of pressure increased and my baby was born 10 minutes later!
>
> *Kate, mum of one*

127

Pushing stage

This is it: the past 40-odd weeks are almost over and you're about to meet your baby for the first time! If you haven't had an epidural the only way to describe the second stage is like needing to do a massive poo. Someone once said to me it felt like she was 'vomiting out of her bum'! What she meant was that there is no way you can hold back; your body is amazing and literally wants to expel your baby by pushing down on all your nerves in your bottom. Getting into a deep squat, on to a birthing stool or on your knees are the perfect positions to get pushing: no one can go for a poo lying on their back. With every contraction you need to work with your body and push your baby's head down into your pelvic floor. Sometimes it takes practice, so don't worry if you don't get it at first – your midwife will help you. They may use a torch and mirror to see if they can see your baby's head and help you to push in the right place. You may want to put your finger inside to feel how close your baby's head is to being born: trust me, giving birth is not about dignity. As your baby is close to being born you may feel a hot, burning sensation as the widest part of the head stretches the skin around your vagina and perineum. This is when all that perineal massage really pays off and hopefully your baby's head stretches that skin without causing any tearing.

So some tips for pushing include:

- Get into any upright position – gravity is your friend!
- Work with your body – this is it, you're almost there.
- Every push brings your baby lower and closer to being born – don't give up.
- Remember to breathe slowly as the head is being born (or crowns); it will allow the skin to stretch and not tear.
- You can ask for a warm compress, such as a flannel on your perineum, to ease the burning sensation.

Third stage

You've done it! All that hard work and your wet, squishy baby is out! They may not be pink straight away – that's normal – a few good cries and all that oxygen will turn their skin to a healthy colour. They may be covered in white cream called vernix, which is the amazing moisturiser that has kept their skin in perfect condition while they've lived in water for the past nine months. Keeping them skin-to-skin with you (or your partner) is a lovely way to keep them warm, regulate their breathing and calm them down.

As this is all going on your midwife will keep a close eye on your bleeding. It's now recommended that babies' cords are left attached, to pulsate, which basically means the blood flowing from the placenta to the baby isn't cut off with a clamp as that extra oxygenated blood is so important for your baby. Your midwife may recommend you have an injection of a hormone called syntocinon into your thigh to help contract your uterus and help your placenta come out. You may, however, decide not to have this injection and opt for a natural delivery of the placenta. It's best to be open-minded about this and see what your midwife advises at the time.

Either way, the best news about your placenta – it's soft! It will literally just fall out with some gentle pulling on the cord, and it's like a large piece of liver. Don't worry if you don't want to see it – lots of people aren't keen, but you may be surprised at how amazing it is – after all, it has kept your baby alive for 40 weeks! Your partner may want to look at it or photograph it, so you can look at it later when you're feeling a bit more normal. Some people choose to keep their placenta – to eat, encapsulate (freeze-dried and made into tablets) or bury in the garden. You can pretty much do what you want with it, so discuss with your partner in advance. If you do choose to take it home it's best to have a large plastic box with a lid to carry it in.

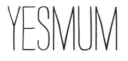

YESMUM

HOLLIE DE CRUZ, LONDON HYPNOBIRTHING AND @THEYESMUMMUM

Preparing for the birth of your baby can be a daunting time, both physically and mentally. But it's important to remember that you are a strong and capable woman! A quick and easy way to start thinking more positively is to start each day with some powerful affirmations.

This simple habit can have an amazing transformative effect on your mindset. Write down your favourite positivity quotes or buy a pack of cards with inspiring affirmations already written on them, and then keep them by your bed, in your handbag, anywhere within reach so that whenever you are having a wobble, you can pick a new card and read it aloud and embrace an encouraging message.

Calmness, confidence and self-belief are great for dealing with those tricky moments during pregnancy, and when you come to the actual birth, you can recall all of those positive thoughts you've had during your pregnancy.

Each affirmation acts like a tiny fist-pump to yourself: a reminder that YOU CAN DO THIS! So go, mama!

I put all fear aside
as I prepare for the
birth of my baby.

I take control of
what I can, and let
go of what I can't.

BIRTH STORY: HOME BIRTH

ANNALISE, FIRST BABY

I had never known that a home birth was an option for us before we discussed the birth with our midwife. The thought of being in hospital gave me the willies; I have a phobia of both me and other people being sick, so a labour ward was the sort of place I wanted to give a wide berth (excuse the pun). The thought of taking that anxiety out of labour was the initial appeal, but quickly other pros mounted up, and all I kept thinking was that we could change our minds at any point and go into hospital if we wanted. Planning a home birth gave us a choice.

When I first mentioned a home birth to my husband, Guy, he was against the idea. He was worried about the possibility of something going wrong. Both our fathers are retired doctors and were sceptical, which added to his hesitancy. I kept reminding him that we could transfer to the hospital at any point – we weren't ruling anything out. It took a few weeks of mulling it over, but eventually Guy came round to the idea, supporting my decision.

Guy and I spent a lot of time preparing for the birth: Guy looked after the logistics, working out how to set up the pool and find the right adaptor for our taps. I focused on getting myself in the right physical condition and mindset. I was doing lots of exercise, such as yoga, swimming, step and resistance training. I was also doing my pelvic-floor exercises and perineum massage. I listened to a hypnobirthing track as I went to sleep at night, and also found it really useful in helping me get back to sleep when I was struck with insomnia.

SUNDAY 12 OCTOBER 2014
1:27 a.m.

I was five days past my due date when I felt my first contraction. I woke up at 1:27 a.m. to a strong tightening in my stomach that faded away. I lay still, wondering what would happen next, and shortly after felt the same sensation rising and falling.

I slipped out of bed, not wanting to wake up Guy, and went to lie down on the sofa. I put on my hypnobirthing track, taking the opportunity to nap between contractions, which at this point were around 8 minutes apart. After two 40-minute loops of the

132

track, the contractions were getting stronger so I put on a DVD of *Cold Feet*, one of my favourite TV series, to distract me and moved on to my birthing ball. As the contractions came, I rested my head on the arm of the sofa, rolled my hips on the ball and closed my eyes. I had set myself the target of 6 a.m. to wake Guy. When 6 a.m. arrived, I still felt pretty relaxed, so I decided to hold out for another hour. Just after 7 a.m., I went into our bedroom, nudged Guy gently and whispered, 'Guy, the baby's coming.' His eyes burst open and he leapt up. 'Really? Where? Now?'

Once Guy had properly woken up, I updated him on the past hours. Together we timed a couple of contractions, had some breakfast, got showered and dressed and at 9 a.m. paged our midwife to let her know that our baby was ready.

The midwife on call called us back soon afterwards. We chatted about my progress and how I was feeling, 'That all sounds great,' she said reassuringly. 'Keep doing what you're doing – lots of walking around and moving – and give me a call again when the contractions are three minutes apart, and really strong, so strong you can't think or talk through them.' Before putting down the phone, she said, 'Each time a contraction comes, say to yourself "bring it on". The bigger and stronger, the more you're progressing.' It was a piece of advice that carried me through the labour.

We called our immediate families to let them know that we were on, and were brought to tears by a call with Guy's mother, who explained that she'd secretly hoped that the baby would make an appearance today as it was the 12th anniversary of the death of her father, our baby's great-grandfather, a very special man.

9:30 a.m.

It was a beautiful, sunny, autumnal Sunday morning, so Guy and I headed out to our local park for a walk. We picked up coffees and walked slowly around our favourite wildlife garden, talking about our baby, its names and our hopes and dreams for him or her. Guy was keeping track of the contractions and would say, 'You should be having a contraction around n—', and on cue I would feel one rising.

After about an hour of walking, the contractions had increased in intensity and we headed home. Along the way the contractions would stop me in my tracks and I would

133

contraction, I remember a young family passing us, smiling and giving us the thumbs-up. Once home, we attached the TENS machine. I returned to the birthing ball and Guy started setting up the birthing pool in the back room of our flat. The contractions were coming every 3 minutes, but I could still think and talk through them so knew I just needed to keep going – Guy and I would count together (he'd call from the back of the flat) so I knew how long until it would pass; I knew when we reached 20 seconds that it was going to ease again.

11 a.m.

Around 11 a.m. the contractions reached such an intensity that we decided to call the midwife. The midwife explained to Guy that she was up at the hospital with a new mother (her first delivery of the day) and that she'd be with us within the hour. When I opened the door to her, it was a huge relief and I burst into tears.

Our midwife was fantastic. She walked in, sat me down and chatted to me about how I was feeling, watched a couple of contractions, checked the baby's and my heart rates, and then examined me. 'You're 3cm dilated. I'm going to stay.' The golden words; I was so relieved.

From this point it was all about progress, 'bringing on' the contractions. I'd been sitting on my birthing ball, rotating my hips, using my TENS machine and breathing to relax through the contractions (pursing my lips and breathing out 'golden spirals'), but to get things going, I needed to move around. I got to my feet and started pacing up and down our hallway, looking for places to lean on as the contractions washed through me.

Guy had just served our midwife some lunch when her phone rang. My ears pricked up when I heard her say, 'I'll be with you in five minutes, I'm just around the corner.' The midwife put down the phone and said to Guy, 'There's a lady round the corner pushing with her second child. I'm afraid I have to go. You'll understand when you have a second child. I'll be back as soon as the other midwife on call gets there.' And she ran out the door.

There was nothing else to do but carry on as we were doing. I continued pacing while Guy started filling the pool. I remained calm for around 45 minutes before I started longing for her return. I sat myself at the front window and gazed out at the road, squinting at every car that passed, asking Guy, 'Is that her?'

3 p.m.

Within the hour, she was back. This time, when she walked in, she was wearing a smock and carrying lots of bags of medical paraphernalia. I thought to myself, 'This is more like it!' Our midwife had reached the other house five minutes before the baby had arrived – her second delivery of the day. The second midwife had arrived shortly afterwards, having had to hitch-hike a lift in a police van (a story in itself). It was an extraordinary day for our midwives.

The midwife carried out more checks and suggested I get in the shower for a change of scenery. I stepped into the shower and got down on all fours, and what a relief it was. Initially, I thought that the shower was slowing down my progress as the contractions eased, but it was actually relief from the warm water. I remained there for what I thought was 30 minutes, but was actually 2 hours. Guy kept popping his head round but I just apologetically asked him to leave me. I felt very calm and just wanted to be alone and focus on the contractions. The midwife intermittently, quietly and discreetly, came in and checked our heart rates. Hearing the little heartbeat of my baby was amazing. It was a constant reminder to me that this was a team effort, I was not alone. My little baby was going through something even bigger than me and remaining calm. I was so proud.

6 p.m.

At around 6 p.m., I asked the midwife what my options were. I felt like I was having contractions that seemed to go on and on, running into each other. I was disappointed that my waters hadn't broken and I was worried it was holding my progress back. The midwife suggested another examination and then to get into the pool. The examination confirmed I was progressing well and had reached 7cm. She described my waters as 'bulging'.

7 p.m.

I made my way down to our back room, where Guy had created the most beautiful space around the pool with candles and music. As soon as I saw the water I virtually dived in. As I submerged, a contraction took over me, and at the same time I felt my waters pop. The midwife tucked herself discreetly to my left and Guy to my right. The midwife left Guy to do the encouraging while she wrote up my notes and calmly answered questions and monitored everything. About an hour later I started feeling the urge to push. At first I didn't really know what I was doing but after a few attempts the midwife suggested I keep my voice low and explained that I had strong but short contractions so to really try and drag them out. Guy was incredible: encouraging me, filling up my water bottle and reminding me to drink, filling up the pool with warm water and keeping so calm. He went through waves of emotions; laughing, crying and quietly just absorbing the atmosphere. I remember it being dark and very calm – probably because I mostly had my eyes closed. I felt very safe, focused and supported.

9 p.m.

After an hour of bearing down I was tired. I had only eaten a piece of toast and my energy stores were getting low. Guy knelt beside me and said, your next push is going to be for Poppy (my niece). As the contraction rose I thought of Poppy's little face and I found a new strength. Next up was my grandmother, followed by Guy's grandfather (whose anniversary it was) and it carried on.

Shortly afterwards we were joined by our second midwife. This arrival was another huge help: I knew I must be getting close if back-up was arriving. I remember feeling something, like a little nose nudging; one more push and the baby crowned. My immediate reaction was to leap out the water and jump up and down, but the midwives told me to breathe and listen very carefully as I needed to do some very small pushes to avoid tearing. I followed their instruction and felt the head deliver. I remember looking down between my legs and seeing a torch light flashing around. The midwife told Guy to join her and showed him our baby's face in a hand mirror – its little eyes blinking and head looking around.

9:28 p.m.

With the next and final contraction I pushed the rest of the body out. I reached down and lifted my baby up in front of me. The midwives spotted that the cord had got tangled around the baby's neck, so they both quickly jumped in and unwound it. I then lifted the baby out the water. 'It's a girl,' I announced, followed by, 'and she looks like your dad, Guy.' In the background INXS's 'Beautiful Girl' was playing. It was a moment of my life that I will never forget.

I sat back into the water and the midwives placed my daughter in my arms and latched her on to feed – her body submerged in the pool to keep warm, with a little hat on her head and a towel over her shoulders. Once all the goodness had been pumped from the placenta, Guy stepped forward and cut the cord, separating my little baby and me for the first time. We sat for 20 minutes while the midwives filled out the paperwork and made a round of tea. Guy took our daughter for some skin-to-skin and I stayed in the pool while we waited for signs that the placenta had detached. After 45 minutes, the midwife stoked up an injection to speed up the process and as I stood up to have it administered, I spotted drops of blood in the water. With one final push (I really didn't think I had it in me), I delivered it!

11:30 p.m.

By 11:30 p.m. our wonderful midwives had weighed our daughter, administered a vitamin K injection into her little leg, completed the paperwork, cleared up the placenta and were ready to go. Our daughter was the third baby they had delivered that day – they are superhumans. We thanked them for everything (how do you even start to thank people who have just done what they did?), and I took our baby to our bed, where we rested and fed. Guy emptied the birthing pool – with a whisky – and when it was all cleared joined us in bed. Just the three of us; our new, wonderful family.

PAIN RELIEF

WHAT YOU REALLY NEED TO KNOW TO MAKE AN INFORMED DECISION

Knowing about TENS, epidural and other pain-relief options ahead of the birth can help you make confident decisions. Remember to stay open-minded: you make the choices that are right for you at the time.

TENS (Transcutaneous Electrical Nerve Stimulation)
A TENS machine sends mild electrical impulses to your back via electrode pads that stick to your skin. You remain in control of the strength of the pulses, which can be varied, using the controls on the machine. The TENS machine is essentially a form of pain relief but it doesn't involve any pharmaceuticals, so has no effect on your baby and also means you are able to be fully present and not left feeling out of control in any way. The electrical pulse it produces stimulates the body to produce endorphins, which are the body's natural pain relief. If you use the TENS machine from early on in labour you're essentially filling your body with endorphins, meaning you can enjoy a more comfortable labour, even when everything is established and contractions are coming thick and fast. You can buy or hire a TENS machine, so make sure if you choose to use one you allow for enough time – no one likes a last-minute online panic!
Advantages:
- Portable, so can be used while staying mobile/active.
- Works well in early labour (you can stay at home longer in the first stage).
- No effect on baby.
- You control the strength of the pulse you receive.

Disadvantages:
- You can't use it in the pool (water and electricity don't mix!).

Water/birth pool

A lot of women often ask me if using water in labour means you have to give birth in the pool – well, the answer is absolutely not! Using water can be anything from having a lovely bath in early labour at home, standing in the shower with the shower head onto the bottom of your back or using a birthing pool once in established labour. You can even use the pool for pain relief but deliver your baby out of the water, if that's your preference. Remember to be open-minded. I've looked after women in labour who weren't even sure they liked the idea of using the pool but once they got in they didn't want to get out and ended up having a beautiful water birth. I've also cared for women who used the pool throughout their entire labour and got out at the end and birthed on dry land. Have a chat with your midwife and find out your options. *One study found that only 24 per cent of first-time mothers who had water births needed pain-relieving drugs compared to 50 per cent of those who didn't use water.*

Questions to think about include: does the hospital have birth pools available and if so how many? Most UK midwives should be trained in supporting women who wish to have a water birth, so if your midwife on the day isn't confident, for whatever reason, it's worth asking for another midwife to care for you. If you're thinking about having a home birth it's worth exploring your options for having a pool set up at home. You can hire them or buy them new online, or even purchase second-hand ones – just make sure they're fully sterilised with disinfectant and always use a brand-new sterile liner. You need to check your tap adapters and water pressure. It's not overly complicated, but I've seen some very stressed-out partners trying to fit the hose pipe to their tap via all sorts of methods (gaffer tape, a cake-piping nozzle). It's not what you want while you're in labour, so make sure you know what you're doing well in advance.

> The pool was amazing. The hot water made me feel relaxed and seemed to take the pressure off my back and pelvis. I never wanted to get out.
>
> *Karmel, mum of one*

Advantages:

- Calms you down and reduces anxiety – which lessens your perception of pain and gives you confidence in your ability to give birth. Go, mama!
- Supports your weight and makes it easier for you to stay upright, helping your pelvis to open up so your baby can pass through. The buoyancy of the water also makes it easier to change positions to help with contractions.
- Reduces the risk of tearing. The water softens the tissues of your perineum (see pages 92–3), making them more supple and able to stretch to accommodate your baby's head as it passes through. This also means you're less likely to need an episiotomy.
- Relaxing in warm water helps the production of pain-relieving endorphins.
- You can combine it with other forms of pain relief, including gas and air (see opposite), massage, acupressure and aromatherapy.
- It's peaceful! The pool itself is a quiet, private environment, which helps you feel safe and secure. Some women want their partners in the pool with them or to stay right next to them, supporting them.

> There was no way my husband was getting in the pool with me – not only had I weed in the pool, but the pool was my sacred space, which belonged to me. He was brilliant at holding my hand through the contractions, changing the music and refilling my water bottle.'
>
> *Katie, mum of two*

Disadvantages:

- The water may make you too relaxed and slow your labour down (it's recommended that you're at least 5cm dilated and contracting regularly before you use the pool).
- If there are any reasons why your midwife recommends that your baby's heartbeat is monitored continuously on a CTG machine (e.g. if the baby has pooed during labour). Some hospitals offer wireless monitoring of your baby called telemetry – speak to your midwife for more information.
- You can't use a pool if you have had pethidine or an epidural, although you can have either after leaving the pool.

Gas and air (Entonox)

Gas and air is a mixture of oxygen and nitrous oxide and is breathed in via a mask or mouthpiece. It's available in all hospitals and birth centres and if you're planning a home birth your community midwives will bring it to your home. It won't take away the pain/sensation of the contractions but it will relieve them by making you feel a bit like you've had a few too many gin and tonics. It takes about 15–20 seconds to work, so make sure you start inhaling it at the beginning of the contraction so it's kicked in by the time you reach the peak of the contraction. It takes a few seconds to wear off, which is when you might feel a bit giddy, spaced out or even really giggly (I've seen women in absolute hysterics after using it!).

Advantages:

- It has no side effects for the baby during labour.
- Combined with the pool it can be all you need for pain relief.
- It's very accessible – you can use it in the bath, pool or shower as the pipe is relatively long.
- In hospital it never runs out! (At home the midwives will have a supply of canisters but may need to get more from the hospital.)

Disadvantages:

- It may make you feel sick (however this is often the effects of labour), but you can stop using it straight away if this is the case.
- Some women don't like the sensation of feeling 'high' or the tingly sensation it can give.

Opiates, e.g. pethidine, morphine, diamorphine, meptid

An opiate drug is usually given via an injection in the top of the thigh or in the bottom and takes about 20 minutes to fully take effect. As it has to be prescribed by a doctor, it's not always available in every hospital, so it's worth checking with your midwife beforehand. As it can make you feel nauseous, your midwife may recommend having an anti-sickness drug at the same time.

Advantages:

- If you've had a very long latent phase of labour (the early stage) and have not slept it can be used to help you relax and sleep – some labours are

stalled due to tiredness, which means the cervix doesn't dilate effectively.
- You can still have an active birth and don't have to be continuously monitored.

Disadvantages:
- It can make you feel woozy, sick and sometimes forgetful and confused.
- It crosses the placenta, so if given too close to delivery it can cause breathing problems for the baby (your midwife might recommend that a neonatal doctor is present for delivery in case of this).
- It can interfere with the baby's first feed due to making the baby sleepy and therefore difficult to feed.

Epidurals

Epidurals get a lot of negative press so it's only fair to be honest about them and give a balanced view. Although I've never personally had one, I've looked after hundreds of women who have had one, and who have had a positive birth experience.

An epidural is the only form of pain relief available in labour that will give you full relief from the contractions. It's administered by an anaesthetist by passing a thin tube (via a needle) into a space in your back. The needle is then taken away and the tube is held in place with lots of sticky tape so it won't come out. It works by numbing the nerves that carry pain signals from the brain to your uterus so you can still move your legs, although they may feel heavy and numb.

As you are less likely to feel the sensation to go for a wee (emptying the bladder is really important during labour) it is recommended that you have a catheter inserted into your urethra via a small tube. This may feel a bit uncomfortable so your midwife won't put it in until your epidural is working effectively. This then stays in for at least 12 hours after your baby has been born. As epidurals can sometimes make your blood pressure drop, it's also recommended you have some fluids via an IV (intravenous) drip. This is usually a saline drip but you can still drink fluids as well. (Nothing too heavy, though – water, coconut water and energy drinks are good options). You will need to be continuously monitored on a CTG machine throughout labour.

I got the chance to actually get a breather after hours of back-to-back contractions. If like me you're having a long labour, an epidural provides a lot of people with much-needed respite after no sleep. Timed right, it gives you the break to recharge, and to push at the final leg.

Nada, mum of two

Advantages:
- It can give really good long-term pain relief for labour.
- Excellent if you're exhausted and need a rest and some sleep.
- It can be brilliant if you're experiencing all your labour in your back and nothing else has helped relieve this.

Disadvantages:
- Epidurals can slow down labour as you're most likely to be in one or two positions on the bed; therefore you may need a hormone drip called Syntocinon to help give those contractions a boost.
- You're more likely to need an assisted delivery (instrumental delivery), especially if this is your first baby, as it's harder to push with an epidural on board. This will either be by a ventouse (a small cup placed on the baby's head) or forceps. Both are carried out by an obstetric doctor.
- If you do have an instrumental delivery (depending on if you've had a baby vaginally before), you are more likely to need an episiotomy to make space for the baby's head.
- About 1 in 100 women experience a postural puncture headache with an epidural and you may need to go to theatre for a blood patch.
- The medication used with an epidural can make your skin itchy – this can be relieved by medication given by your midwife.
- You may have a sore back for a few days after your baby is born – however this can also be associated with pregnancy and labour itself.

So there you have it; all you need to know about pain relief for labour/birth. Keep an open mind about what's right for you. Labour can be unpredictable and there are no medals for who did it with or without drugs. It's about having a positive birth, which might be with just a whiff of gas and air.

ENGAGING YOUR SENSES

When we're in strange places with people we don't know our bodies trigger our fight-or-flight response. This stimulates the production of adrenalin and means our birthing muscles stop getting the blood and oxygen they need to work comfortably and efficiently. Creating an environment that feels more private and homely will help reassure you that you are safe and that no one is observing you (we're very primal when it comes to birth).

A few little extras, whether you're planning a birth at home or in hospital, can really help you relax. Remember you need all the oxytocin you can get during labour. Oxytocin is the 'love' hormone and is needed to initiate and maintain labour. It requires a dark, quiet, familiar, non-threatening environment in order to flow. If you're having your baby in hospital, it's likely you're going to encounter the smell of bleach or hand-gel, so it's a good idea to override that with your own comforting scents. I'm a big fan of essential oils – they are easy to use and incredibly effective during pregnancy and birth, when your sense of smell is heightened. My favourites include:

- Lavender: Well known to aid relaxation and promote calm. Also a painkiller that stimulates circulation and healing and may strengthen contractions.
- Clary sage: One of the oils that you should avoid during pregnancy until 37 weeks, but fine once you're in labour, clary sage can strengthen contractions. It's also a great oil for lifting your spirits and reducing anxiety.
- Peppermint: A generally uplifting and refreshing oil.
- Chamomile: Soothes, calms and helps to reduce tensions and anxiety.
- Jasmine: Acts as a uterine tonic, painkiller and anti-spasmodic. Also known to strengthen contractions and can be used to aid delivery of the placenta.

During my third labour I inhaled clary sage and lavender on a cold wet flannel every time I got a contraction. It was seriously powerful and got me through the toughest parts, as lavender is a muscle relaxant and sedative and clary sage boosts contractions. Winning combo!

PUSH MUSIC

Creating a playlist of songs that make you feel happy and safe is a really lovely way as a couple to think about your birth (and a fun way to have a giggle at some of your old CDs collecting dust).

Music has the power to make you feel all sorts of emotions, and you certainly will go through many in labour! It doesn't need to be whale music and pan pipes – any music you had at your wedding or remember from childhood, for instance, is likely to bring up those nostalgic, emotive memories and associations of feeling loved and at ease. Mix it up: maybe have some instrumental pieces when you want to feel focused and in your zone, and then some up-tempo stuff for moments when you want to feel more energised and alive. Basically, the more you can appeal to all of your senses with positive triggers, the better! You may want to pack some small portable speakers in your hospital bag as not every hospital/birth centre will have access to a music player.

Latent phase/first stage: The time when you'll be mostly at home relaxing. So think chill-out tunes. You may want to consider listening to these via some headphones in the bath, snoozing in between the milder contractions. Remember, you don't want to be using up all your energy at this stage, so get in the zone and try to stay relaxed.

Active phase: Something a little more upbeat could be really great here. I have seen (and have done it myself) women dancing to the beat of music during this stage of labour. Imagine sitting on the birthing ball, rocking your hips from side to side to a great tune with a great bass. Your partner might get involved too, and even your midwife!

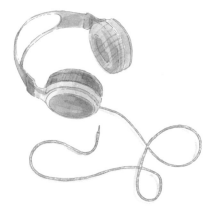

STAND AND DELIVER

POSITIONS FOR LABOUR

I often hear women telling me their birth stories, and a common theme comes through: 'I had to get on the bed to have monitoring' or 'the midwife/doctor needed to listen to the baby's heartbeat so I got on the bed.'

There is no rule written in any guideline/hospital policy that says a woman has to be on the bed for monitoring. If it is advised that it is safer to monitor your baby's heartbeat during labour with a CTG machine then ask to stand, lean over the bed or sit on a ball, because this is your labour and you know the benefits of staying upright. Remember UFO! (See page 123). Get your birth partner to ask for the bed to be moved, for a birthing ball (or take your own in) or for birthing mats to be put down on the floor. Any unnecessary equipment can be moved out of the way to make space for you to be active.

Active birth was first introduced to me as a first-year student midwife 10 years ago. It became something I was so passionate about I even wrote my final-year dissertation on the subject: 'Alternative Positions of the Mother in the Second Stage of Labour'. There have been hundreds of studies written about why staying upright and moving around in labour is more beneficial for the woman. So just to clarify some of the benefits:

Benefits of active birth:
- Shorter, more efficient, labour.
- Help the labouring mum to cope with the intensity of contractions.
- Less risk of fetal distress as there is better blood flow to the placenta.
- Working with gravity rather than against it.
- Partners can give physical support, helping them to get involved.
- Minimal trauma for mum and baby.

Opposite are a few great ideas for keeping active in labour.

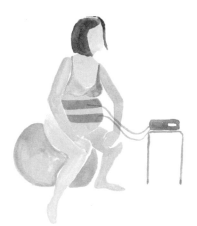
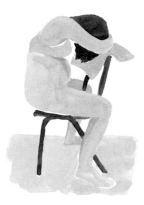
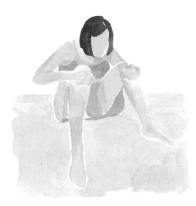
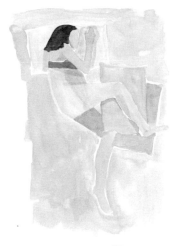
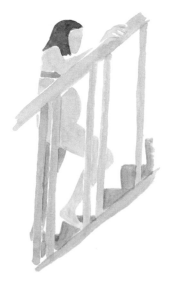
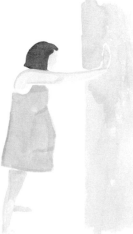

POOING – AND WHY IT'S NORMAL

I think it's one of the most commonly asked questions us midwives hear: 'Will I poo when I'm giving birth?' In fact, 80–90 per cent of women do a poo at some point during labour. And do you know what? Us midwives get a little excited when we see a poo. Seriously, we do, because it often means the baby is getting closer to being born and that is really exciting! But we don't scream and shout 'Look she's done a poo, look everyone!' We quietly and subtly clear it away without anyone (partners included) noticing. I have constructed a list, to dispel all myths about all things poo-related.

- Midwives don't really mind poo. It often means the baby coming, so we get super-excited and slowly start to put our gloves on.
- Life goes on after pooing in front of your partner. You've already been naked, had sex, probably vomited, passed wind etc. in front of them, so a poo is really no biggie.
- As the baby pushes down in your pelvis, it pushes on all the nerves and muscles in your bottom. So if there's some poo in there, then of course it's going to come out. Giving birth really does feel like going for the biggest poo of your life.
- If you can, go for a poo in early labour. Women often have diarrhoea at the onset of labour, which is the body's way of having a clear-out.
- Don't worry about what you have eaten. Depriving yourself of food during early labour because you're worried about pooing is a bad idea. A runner does not prepare for a marathon by starving herself and you shouldn't either. You and your baby need energy to have the endurance for birth.
- 'Bear down' and 'push like you need a poo' are some phrases you may hear us midwives say during birth. Focus on this: get into a position as if you are going to open your bowels, such as a deep squat, all fours or on a birthing stool. No one poos lying down or with their legs in stirrups – so think about this if you're asked to get on the bed to deliver the baby.

STEPH DOUGLAS, DON'T BUY HER FLOWERS

As we arrived at the hospital I was taken in to the assessment room. I could hear nervous whispered conversations from couples sitting quietly behind curtains waiting to see a midwife, all likely to be sent home again because they'd come in too early. I, on the other hand, was pretty far along and was wailing and MOOING like a cow. It's happened in both my labours and it's not even a noise I can do on demand, but it really is the exact sound of a loud and distressed cow.

The midwife was asking me to get up on the bed so she could check how dilated I was, but the contractions were getting closer and closer and I needed to be standing up. On my mum's advice – she was a midwife – I'd hung on at home for as long as possible, which meant I was pretty much good to go on arrival at the hospital. So I kept trying to get up, and then mooing a bit, and getting back off the bed. I was making quite a scene behind my little curtained-off area.

And then it happened: the pressure all got too much and I ripped down my knickers and shat. As I was standing it was from quite a height so – much like a cow-pat, to continue the theme – it splatted all over the floor. Rather than quietly hope no one had heard, I accompanied it with yells of 'I'm shitting, I'm shittiiiing' while my husband patted my back and said 'We know, darling', then I apologised repeatedly to the wall of curtains that must have been hiding horrified couples.

But you know what? I didn't care. I was in labour and I knew that my body was doing what it was supposed to do.

So, is birth beautiful? It is definitely incredible and mind-blowing as well as messy. An actual human being comes out of your body. It still freaks me out a little. And despite what he saw, my husband also remembers it as an awesome thing, watching me do something so incredible and with such determination. So, despite all the crapping and mooing, I suppose it was pretty beautiful.

38 WEEKS

THERE'S A FOOTBALL
IN BETWEEN MY LEGS

YOUR BABY IS ABOUT AS LONG AS A LEEK — NEARLY
50CM (FROM HEAD TO TOE, BUT IT IS CURLED UP
INSIDE YOU) — AND WEIGHS JUST OVER 3KG.

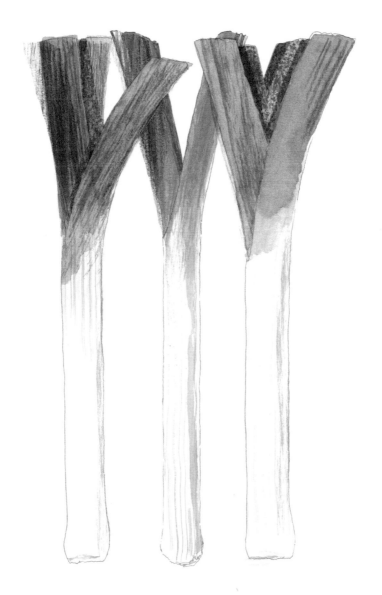

PACKING YOUR HOSPITAL BAG

I've seen a lot of birth-bag checklists in my time, and what always baffles me is – quite frankly – what a load of crap they all are. They seem to be mostly compiled by companies who sell baby products that they want you to buy and put in said birth bag, and as a pregnant woman more concerned with how you're going to birth a human, it can be one of those things that doesn't get much informed thought and ends up as a last-minute panic-bought menagerie of rubbish that (I guarantee) you will not use in labour.

So take a moment to think about the three Ws when it comes to this bag: What's it for? Who's it for? When's it for? The answer is that it's a bag of essentials for YOU to use when YOU'RE in labour, either at home or in hospital. It doesn't need to include your baby's entire wardrobe, however ovary-achingly gorgeous the contents of that might be.

Realistically, if you have a straightforward birth, you are not going to be in hospital for very long after you've had your little one, and if you do have to stay in for longer, your partner or family can always bring you more baby supplies if necessary. What I'm saying is: make this bag about YOU. Think of it as your hand luggage for the best trip you're ever going to take. Your companion for what could be a long-haul flight through multiple time zones.

So I've compiled my list of what I think makes a kick-ass birth bag.

It's also worth me saying that it's essential that your birth partner packs the birth bag. Yes, really. I have seen so many fathers-to-be desperately trying to find a hair band that their partner needs 'NOW' in the bottom of the bag, while flinging out baby blankets, maternity pads and extra-large black cotton knickers. Lay all of this stuff out on your bed so that you remain in control of what's going in, but let your partner pack it, because it's very likely that they're going to be the one navigating the contents in labour, and if they don't know the difference between a sanitary/maternity/breast pad, we're all in trouble. Here goes:

- Home comforts such as a pillow, and not with your best 1,000-thread cotton pillowcase on it. Just a cheapo one will do. Whether you're having your baby at home, in a birth centre or in a hospital, one of the best ways to keep your mind and body at ease is to make your surroundings as familiar and intimate as possible. In strange places with people we don't know (especially places associated with ill health/emergencies) our bodies naturally trigger our fight-or-flight response. This puts us on high alert and on the lookout for danger. It also stimulates the production of adrenalin, which means our birthing muscles stop getting the blood and oxygen they need to work comfortably and efficiently, because their functions are not deemed essential for our survival.
- Lavender oil. This is an all-rounder essential oil, for massage during labour, putting on your maternity pad to help perineal healing and on to your pillow to help with relaxation and sleep. You may also want to include grapefruit as it's uplifting and clary sage to increase contractions (note clary sage should not be used before 37 weeks of pregnancy – see page 144).
- A hot water bottle or wheat bag. Both of these were fantastic for me in early labour when I wanted something on my lower back and pelvis but it was too soon to use the pool.
- A mirror. I really wanted to see the baby's head crowning when I was in the pool, but for the rest of you who aren't so mental it's good to have on hand to check your reflection before the in-laws arrive to meet the new baby.
- A wide head band. This was great for getting my fringe off my face when I felt hot in labour.
- Ridiculously comfy clothes. And by that I mean the most comfortable clothes you have worn in your entire life. Think loose-fitting, soft materials – maybe a nice winceyette shirt that you can button/unbutton depending on temperature. Two tips here: go for something dark, and buy men's so that

you're not obstructed by anything tight-fitting. Perfect for breastfeeding in and if you have a C-section it's not going to irritate your wound.

- Warm socks or slippers. Weirdly, feeling cold is also very normal in labour and putting these on while I was still walking around the room before getting into the pool made me feel cosy. Hospital floors can be a bit chilly on the toes.
- A bikini top if you want to wear one in the pool (you probably won't, but...).
- I'd also suggest taking a lightweight gown/robe. Hospitals are roughly the temperature of the sun, so I'd avoid anything too heavy or fleecy, but you might want something to throw on if you're getting in/out of the pool.
- An iPod with all your playlists on it. Most delivery rooms have CD players, but I really liked having the headphones on my ears during labour and blocking out the sounds around me. Remember to include songs that make you feel happy and safe.
- A really good lip balm that you or your birth partner can easily apply. All that breathing and gas and air can make your lips super-dry.
- Facial moisture spray. This can be in the form of a ready-bought product or as simple as water in a spray bottle. Either way I felt really hot in various stages of my birth and my husband used this on my face and neck to cool me down.
- Earplugs to block out the sound of your annoying partner (only joking!). The post-natal ward is notoriously noisy at night with other babies crying, so these might help you catch a few seconds' sleep.
- Incontinence pants with a built-in pad. They may resemble an adult nappy, but I promise after three births these were the best things I ever wore for the first few days. (Expect to bleed like a really heavy period for a few days.)
- Dark chocolate. I ate the entire bar just after my daughter was born; it was like little squares of heaven and it's full of iron, so a fantastic way to increase your iron levels without feeling guilty!

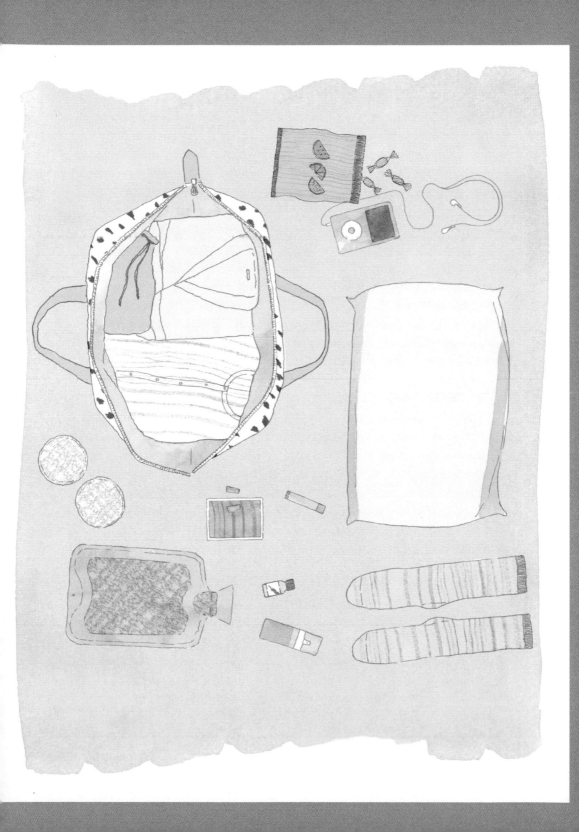

BREECH – A BUM DEAL

During your pregnancy your baby will have been wriggling around and getting into all sorts of positions – transverse, head down, legs down, bum down – all of which are completely irrelevant and us midwives don't worry about it until around now. Most babies by around 36–37 weeks of pregnancy will settle into the head-down position (the head is the largest and heaviest part of the baby), ready for birth. However, around 3 per cent of babies will not play ball and think the breech position (bottom first) is far more comfortable. You may have had a sneaky suspicion that your baby was breech by the hard head pressing into your ribs or the very odd and sometimes painful sensation of kicks on to your bladder or on to your cervix (which I named 'fanny daggers' during my pregnancy with the twins!)

Usually detected by your midwife's skilful palpation of your bump during your antenatal appointment, a breech baby poses some questions and discussions that you may not have considered. If your midwife believes your baby is in the breech position they will recommend you go to the hospital for a 'presentation scan', which simply means a doctor or sonographer will scan you and look at exactly what position your baby is in. This is a good opportunity for you to ask as many questions as possible so you feel well informed and can make the right decision for you and your baby.

IS THERE ANYTHING I CAN DO TO TURN MY BABY?

There isn't much evidence to say that any of these techniques work, but they are thought to be totally harmless, so it's worth giving them a shot.
- Get upside down. You could try kneeling on your bed with your knees comfortably apart and your hip joints over your knees, then rest your

shoulders down on the pillow. Some midwives recommend that this 'knee-chest' position is adopted regularly towards the end of pregnancy, for about 15 minutes, two to three times a day.

- Get burning. Moxibustion (moxa) is a traditional Chinese medicine used to try to turn breech babies. It uses a moxa stick, which looks like a big cigar, on an acupuncture point on the body. This is usually between the toes for breech presentation. When the herbal stick is burned, it should encourage your baby to move and hopefully turn from breech (bottom first) to cephalic (head first). It will certainly increase your baby's movements, if nothing else!
- Get pricking. Moxa alone may not do the job – so combining it with a few sessions of acupuncture from a certified acupuncturist may be more effective. Contact the British Acupuncture Council for more information.

ZOE, MUM OF TWO

I cried when I was told my baby was breech. I had decided that the worse thing (ever) would be to become a mother without ever experiencing even a teeny tiny contraction, let alone to have a caesarean. It just wasn't part of 'the plan'. But I'd watched many ECVs (external cephalic version, where a doctor manually turns the baby) as a midwife, supported women and been amazed at what was possible. I booked myself in without hesitation for the following week.

However, I was determined that I would try and 'turn' the baby myself and spent many an hour with my head hanging off my sofa, being poked at by the acupuncturist, and stunk out our flat with moxibustion, leading to our neighbours upstairs enquiring whether

I had a pregnancy craving for incense sticks! On the instructions it says you should feel 'mild discomfort', and I decided that if I held them there for longer they would work better. The reality was me holding out till I shouted 'too much, STOP' to my husband as I felt my toes burning... It didn't work.

So I went along to my appointment for an ECV in my local hospital. By the time I was lying on a hospital bed waiting for the medication to work to relax my uterus, I had also made peace with having a caesarean so that whatever happened (if the ECV didn't work) I knew it was going to be great anyway (after all, I was going to be a mum and hold my baby very soon!).

I was so chuffed when the naughty little piglet turned! A wonderful forward roll was perfectly performed by the obstetrician and we saw all of this on the ultrasound screen – it was amazing! I hugged the consultant (and felt rather embarrassed after for doing so) and asked him if he prefers red or white wine as I felt he definitely deserved a bottle!

It always makes me sad, though, when I hear someone say they 'had' to have a caesarean because they heard an ECV was horrible and didn't want to do it. Someone is turning your baby and there are sensations that go with that, but having now experienced contractions (twice) it was no way near comparable. The 'worst' bit was getting her out of my pelvis, but I used it as an opportunity to practise my labour breathing and spent most of the ECV imagining I was on a beach in New Zealand, where we had spent our honeymoon the year before.

I feel really lucky that I had the opportunity to turn Charlotte. I'm sat here now with an almost three-year-old and a two-month-old son after two lovely straightforward births and without it my birthing experience would have been very different.

AND WHAT IF NONE OF THESE THINGS WORK?

Despite all your best efforts your baby may not want to budge out of the breech position. It's worth making sure you have an in-depth discussion with your midwife and obstetrician about your options at this stage. Sadly, here in the UK, midwives have lost their skill of delivering a vaginal breech due to the majority of women opting for an elective C-section. This may make you feel less confident in planning a vaginal birth.

Remember that everything is your choice. You may want to consider speaking to and hiring an independent midwife, who may be more skilled and experienced in delivering breech babies. You would need to pay for their services (approximately £2,000–£4,000 just for the birth.) However, if you do decide to go for a vaginal birth, you will be fully supported by your midwives and obstetrician and a detailed birth plan with be made with you. A Supervisor of Midwives may also be involved to ensure you're fully informed on the decisions you make.

When making your decision, remember BRAIN: Benefits, Risks, Alternatives, Instinct, and what if you do Nothing.

If you do decide that having a C-section is the right decision for you and your baby, it can be just as positive and empowering an experience as having a vaginal birth – it's the day you get to meet your baby, after all! Speak to your midwife about having things like the drape lowered as the baby is born, skin-to-skin in theatre and delayed cord clamping. (See pages 61 and 121.)

Useful links:
www.nhs.uk/conditions/pregnancy-and-baby/pages/breech-birth.aspx
www.nct.org.uk/birth/breech-birth

WHAT TO EXPECT IF YOU'RE HAVING A C-SECTION

Sometimes having to let go of plan A and accepting plan B is hard to deal with, especially when it comes to your birth. The truth is, the best birth exists in so many forms, so if it's been recommended that having a C-section is the safest option for you and your baby then let's make it the BEST C-section ever! There are many reasons why it may be recommended that you have an elective section. These include:

- You've already had a caesarean section, and there were complications during the procedure.
- Your baby is in a bottom-down (breech) position, and external cephalic version (ECV) isn't recommended, or hasn't been successful (see pages 157–8).
- You are expecting twins, or more, and the first baby isn't in a head-down position.
- Your baby is in a sideways (transverse) position, or keeps changing their position (unstable lie).
- You have severe pre-eclampsia or eclampsia, and having your baby by vagina will take too long to be safe.
- You have a low-lying placenta (placenta praevia).
- You have a medical condition, such as a certain type of heart disease.
- You've asked to have a caesarean, perhaps because of a previous traumatic vaginal birth.

Whatever the reason, you may understandably be feeling anxious, disappointed, scared, but hopefully excited that you have a date when you will meet your baby! Remember that a positive and safe birth is the most important thing here. A caesarean section is not just a statistic, or a failed natural birth, or life-saving surgery, it's a baby's birth, and a woman's birth into motherhood too.

Once you've met with an obstetrician to discuss the procedure, you will be given a date when your C-section will be performed. During this appointment it's important that you ask any questions that you have or place any special requests, e.g. Can I bring in my own music to be played in theatre? Is my birth partner allowed to take photos? Can I have skin-to-skin with my baby as soon as he or she is born?

You will be given a date and time for when to come into hospital (there are usually three to four elective sections performed each day), but you may not know until the day what number you are on the list. On the day you will get a chance to meet the anaesthetist and discuss the spinal anaesthesia that will be used to make sure you can't feel any pain during the operation. You will also have a midwife with you during the operation and they will be the one helping you with caring for your baby. When it's time for your op, you will be fitted with gorgeous surgical stockings and a hospital gown that opens at the back to allow for the anaesthetist to access your back. It's a good idea to take a camera into theatre to have some lovely photos taken, and a cotton hat for your baby – theatres are a bit on the chilly side and us midwives like to keep babies really warm when they're born.

Remember to remove nail varnish the night before, take off any jewellery and if you are smart SHAVE YOUR OWN PUBIC HAIR – hospital razors are not pleasant. Your midwife will take you and your birth partner into theatre. There are likely to be a large number of people in the operating theatre with you, sometimes up to ten. The staff may include: a midwife; two obstetricians, a theatre nurse and an assistant; an anaesthetist and an assistant.

You will then begin to have the spinal put in by the anaesthetist (usually sitting on the edge of the theatre table) and that takes about 20 minutes to take effect. It doesn't hurt beyond a sharp scratch when the needle goes in. They then poke your legs to check when it's worked and spray cold water on you to check you can't actually feel anything before starting the operation. Once that is working well the midwife will put a catheter into your urethra that will stay in usually until the next morning. You may then experience shivering as the drugs work into your body. You will also have a drip in your hand so that the anaesthetist can give you fluids and drugs if needed.

Your birth partner will sit at the head end, usually with the anaesthetist on the other side of you. (He or she will make jokes about letting you know when they have started when the baby is already half out). A screen will be placed near your head so you can't see what is happening. You shouldn't feel any pain at all during the operation, though you may be aware of some sensations. Some women describe the feeling as 'like having someone doing the washing-up in your tummy'. Five minutes later the baby is delivered and you can ask for the screen to be lowered as the baby is being lifted out (don't worry, you won't actually see the incision).

Depending on how you're feeling you can have skin-to-skin with your baby in theatre or you may prefer your partner to. The doctors remove your placenta and then stitch up your wound with one long continuous piece of thread (you're not really aware of this going on as you'll be staring at this little human you grew for nine months). Mama, you're amazing! You'll then be taken to the recovery bay to have time with your baby and enjoy the best-tasting cup of NHS tea you'll ever have!

It's worth remembering that even though approximately 26 per cent of births last year were via C-section*, it is still major abdominal surgery, so be prepared to take it really, really easy afterwards. Women often say to me that they didn't realise how physically full-on having a C-section would be, even an elective one. You will heal better in the long run if you take it slow in the beginning. Some good tips include:

• Have family members around to help with cooking and cleaning (especially if you have other children to consider).
• Get all your food delivered.
• Only wear big knickers and the loosest of trousers or a long nightshirt.

- Use a maternity pad in your knickers pressed against your scar to keep the area dry.
- Get in some arnica (brilliant for bruising) and Spatone (an iron supplement).
- Lots and lots of rest when you can.
- Don't be a hero! Take the drugs prescribed to you.
- Drink plenty of water and eat fibrous foods – you'll be glad of it when you go for your first poo (seems you don't escape the worry of the first post-birth poo whichever way your baby comes out!).

My baby didn't come out of my vagina, but I grew a human and birthed him, and I'm very proud of that. After years of reflection I've come to the happy conclusion that all of us, each and every woman who pushes a baby out of her body, we're all warriors.

Alice, mum of two

Also, remember that even if you have previously had a C-section, there's usually no reason why you can't try for a VBAC (Vaginal Birth After Caesarean) next time. There are a few small risks involved – for example, your doctor will need to keep an eye on your scar to make sure it doesn't look as if it will rupture during labour – but speak to your midwife about your options. It's usually perfectly possible to deliver your baby by VBAC.

* www.hscic.gov.uk/catalogue/PUB19127

BIRTH STORY: ELECTIVE C-SECTION

SARAH, SECOND BABY

Given my first son was 9lbs and both my husband and I are quite tall, we never expected a small baby, but at 36.5 weeks, this babe was already coming in at 8.5lbs. I returned the next week for a follow-up. Bad news. The scan showed even more dramatic growth and they expected a birth weight of over 10lbs. Now that's a big baby. Too big to deliver naturally, since I had previously had a C-section.

In the days that followed I spoke at length with Clemmie about how to make my C-section experience special. We made a plan. My husband was tasked with making a playlist. First time around I had generic radio playing some awful songs. Rob compiled a CD of music that was soothing and special to us. Clemmie made sure I had skin-to-skin contact immediately post-birth and Rob wanted to cut the cord. I also got hold of some hypnobirthing books and MP3 affirmations. It had never even occurred to me that I could use these techniques to keep me calm, relaxed and focused even in a surgical environment.

Thanks to Clemmie's advice I felt good and prepared – even raving it up on the dance floor of our friends' wedding until midnight two days before the C-section!

On the day, I went into hospital feeling calm and happy. I knew I was doing the best thing for me and my baby. Entering the theatre, I was greeted by friendly, familiar faces and my music was playing. I concentrated on my husband, the music and the excitement that we were about to meet our second child. I honestly forgot there was anyone else in the room. Before I knew it, Quinn was born. He weighed in at 11lbs. Now THAT's a big baby!

The consultant had to wrestle him out of my pelvis as he had got well and truly wedged in. She immediately reassured me that I had made the right decision having the C-section as he wouldn't have delivered naturally. That was exactly the right thing to say. I felt relief and acceptance of the experience. The next 45 minutes, the remainder of the operation, was spent in an intimate bubble, just me, my husband and our boy. The room was still full of people, but Clemmie had helped create an environment where we could be together, happy tears, our music and skin-to-skin.

BIRTH STORY: EMERGENCY C-SECTION

CHARLOTTE, FOUNDER OF
MOTHERLAND.NET, FIRST BABY

Despite being a caesarean baby myself, I hadn't even slightly prepared for the possibility of having one. My mum had been 38, with pre-eclampsia; I was 27, fit, and positive I would push this baby out. But then life got in the way and after an unsuccessful induction – I didn't dilate to even a centimetre – four days later, the decision was made that I should have a section. By this time, I was relieved. Labour hadn't been traumatic (in fact, I had hardly felt the contractions that made crashing wave-shapes on the screen beside me), but I was totally and utterly shattered and ready to meet my baby...

Because I hadn't considered a caesarean, I had no idea what to expect. As I entered theatre and was introduced to the many faces in the room – anaesthetists, assistants and a surgeon – I felt shivery, apprehensive. The surgeon asked me what music I'd like to listen to and I heard myself say, 'Whatever helps you concentrate.' Once the anaesthetic took hold, as I clung on to my husband's hand, I began to calm. The staff were so reassuring and jollying that I felt instantly safe and cared for. They all seemed so excited on my behalf, it was hard to believe they do countless deliveries like this each day. They asked my husband if he'd like to stand on my side or theirs for the birth. He opted for mine – though for a second he was bolder and watched our child emerge...

They told us the operation would take around 20 minutes, so I was astonished to watch my baby emerge from my tummy just 4 minutes later. I'd been so convinced I was having a boy I shouted out, 'Where's his willy?' as they held her up before me. As they stitched me back up, I gazed to my left and watched the midwife weigh and wrap my baby, who was 8lbs 4oz, perfectly healthy, and screaming like a banshee. My husband cut the umbilical cord and when they brought her over for the first time, I felt a surge of euphoria, fear and adoration sweep through my body. While they finished the op, I looked between my tiny new daughter and my husband, my mind fizzing with all these new feelings I never knew were stored within me.

FREEZE!

THE CRUMBS SISTERS

Your ankles are swollen, it feels like there's a watermelon balancing on your bladder and all you want to do is sit down and put your feet up. So what do we suggest? Cooking up a storm.

Hold on, hear us out. Cooking may seem difficult now, at the tail end of pregnancy, but in those early days of babyhood it will be even trickier. And luckily, these dishes are super-easy to prepare. Make double quantities, have some for dinner tonight, portion up the rest and pop in the freezer. Just think: soon you'll be enjoying a delicious stew, perhaps with a glass of red wine and the wonderful feeling of having a beautiful newborn baby nearby.

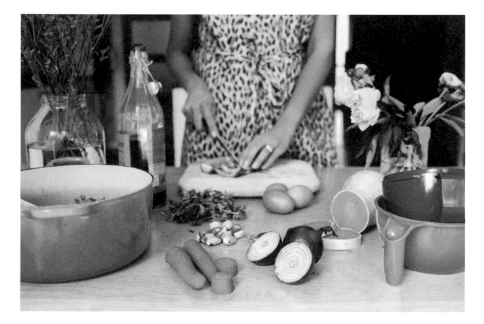

LAMB AND CINNAMON STEW

This is deceptively simple at the same time as being dinner-party worthy. Go on, invite the NCT crew round and impress them (only joking! Keep it all to yourself).

SERVES: *4–5 portions*
START TO FINISH: *10 min prep, 3.5 hours cooking*
1kg diced lamb shoulder (ask your butcher for the bone and throw that in too, for extra flavour)
2 onions, sliced
2 cinnamon sticks
1 tsp dried oregano
olive oil
tin chopped tomatoes
1 litre hot chicken stock
1 glass of white or red wine

1 Put the lamb (and bone, if using), onions, cinnamon, oregano and oil in a large casserole dish or roasting tin. Give it a good stir, so everything is evenly coated. Pop in the oven at 160°C(fan)/180°C/gas mark 4 for an hour, checking and stirring halfway.
2 Pour over the wine, tomatoes and stock and put the casserole lid on. Or if, like me, you don't have one, use tinfoil instead.
3 Return to the oven for two and a half hours. It may sound like a long time, but the lamb is fatty and needs time to melt into the stew.
4 Remove the cinnamon sticks (and bone). Serve with jacket potatoes or roast sweet potatoes. This improves after a couple of days in the fridge (skim the fat off the top before reheating).

To **freeze**: once it has cooled, divide into portions in freezer bags or plastic containers and freeze.

CELERIAC SOUP

The perfect quick lunch to wolf down between baby massage and the local library's Rhyme Time this afternoon – it's all go!

SERVES: *4 portions*
START TO FINISH: *20 mins prep,*
  20 mins cooking
olive oil
1 celeriac, peeled and chopped
2 leeks, finely chopped
water to cover

1 x chicken-stock cube
3 tbsps single cream
A dash of truffle oil – optional
Chopped parsley
2 onions, sliced

1 Splash some olive oil into a large saucepan.
2 Put the pan over a medium heat and throw in the celeriac and leeks.
3 Let them cook for 10 minutes, stirring occasionally.
4 Add enough water to cover the vegetables and crumble in a chicken-stock cube.
5 Give it a stir and bring to the boil.
6 Cover the pan and let it simmer for 20 minutes, until the celeriac is tender.
7 Purée the soup thoroughly, stir in the cream. Season with salt and pepper.
8 Serve with a drizzle of truffle oil and a scattering of parsley.

To freeze: allow to cool and portion into freezer bags or Tupperware.

EIGHT APPLE CAKE

When you have your first child cake takes on a whole new meaning. Suddenly it's a valid meal in itself. This one even has eight apples in it – yum and healthy. Have it for breakfast (with an espresso), have it for tea, with, um, tea. It's a lifesaver.

SERVES: *8 to 12 decent slices*
START TO FINISH: *Just over 1 hour*
  (including peeling and baking)
8 eating apples – peeled, cored and
  chopped (you need about 450g of
  apples)
juice from one lemon
½ tsp ground cinnamon

200g plain flour
1 ½ tsp baking powder
200g caster sugar
3 eggs
6 level tbsps melted butter
1–2 tbsp milk, as needed
one tbsp demerara sugar for topping

1 Heat oven to 180°C; grease and line a 20cm-square cake tin. Toss the apples in the lemon juice and ground cinnamon the minute they're chopped.
2 Combine the rest of the dry ingredients in a bowl. Add the eggs and butter and beat to make a stiff batter. Add milk if it seems a bit dry.
3 Fold the apples (and any remaining lemon juice) into the batter. Pour into the cake tin, smooth down and sprinkle with demerara sugar. Bake for 45 to 50 minutes or until a skewer comes out clean

To freeze: allow to cool, cut into slices, hoover up all the crumbs (yum!) and wrap each individually, very well, in cling film.

HOW YOU MIGHT BE FEELING AND WHY THAT'S OKAY

TIRED

Your body is going through a lot right now. It is having to deal with the extra weight of the baby and all of your organs are in different places. You're mentally, emotionally and physically strained, so feeling tired is completely normal. Make sure you don't try to do too much before the baby comes. You might want to get things ready at home, but remember that getting yourself ready is so much more important for you both.

ANXIOUS

Most women experience anxiety in the lead-up to labour, so know that if you are feeling anxious you are not alone. Try to remember that your body is so capable of this. If you are struggling with anxiety, try some of the following:
- Practise your hypnobirthing breathing (see page 103).
- Ask your partner to massage you (practice makes perfect) (see page 67).
- Make some of those delicious recipes and eat them! (See pages 167/9.)
- Connect with your baby, talk to your bump and tell it how much you can't wait to meet him or her.

EXCITED

As the birth approaches, your excitement steps up a gear, until you turn into the adult equivalent of a five-year-old on Christmas morning. Feeling excited is brilliant: you are about to meet your child! Enjoy your excitement and use its positive energy to help when you are feeling less positive.

Don't forget how amazing you are and what an incredible job you've done so far. You're almost there.

THE 'JUST FOR YOU' LIST

Let's not be unrealistic here, nothing – but nothing – can prepare you for how something weighing around 7lbs and is approximately 50cm long can take up all your time and energy. But I won't divulge too much. So this is the time to really think about you and your needs because it's very easy to be so focused on your baby. Some of the things I did for myself, before the birth, really meant that I felt like I had taken care of the things that were important to me. These were not obvious to my husband but meant I wasn't stressing about them after the birth, and I could really enjoy those first weeks.

Things I bought:

- The comfiest cotton pants known to man. You will be wearing them all day and all night and maternity pads make you feel like a 13-year-old who's just got her period. All the glamour.
- The softest cotton nightshirt. Ideal for hospital and for home as it was long enough to cover my pants but unbuttoned at the front, so gave perfect access for the boobs (which, by the way, need accessing ALL THE TIME).
- Bed socks. Again, lovely to have warm feet when you're resting in bed with a newborn (go for cashmere if you're feeling flush).
- My favourite facial moisturiser. Make-up routines go out of the window when you've just had a baby, mainly because you don't care how you look and also you're high as a kite on oxytocin, sniffing your newborn's head.
- A gorgeous-smelling candle. Sometimes you can't beat the smell of a divinely fragranced home (plus it also hides the smell of nappies).

Things I did:

- Signed up to online food shopping – game-changer moment.
- Got a mani and pedi. In the throes of labour I remember looking down at my perfectly painted, vibrant red nails and feeling chuffed with myself.
- Had a wonderful pregnancy massage. Nothing beats that floaty feeling after being massaged in lovely oils (and then heading home for a nap).

SHIT JUST GOT REAL

When I used to run the local antenatal classes as a community midwife we always ended the morning with an 'ask the midwife' section, allowing couples to ask us, well, just about anything. One question we got asked time and time again was: 'what's the best way to get to the hospital?'

I was working in a busy part of south-east London and the thought of road closures, diversions and London rush hour filled the couples (but mainly the birth partners) with fear.

Hopefully, by now, you will have visited the hospital you're planning on having your baby at – usually when you have your scan or various other midwife appointments. If you live in a city I would always recommend getting a taxi to the hospital when in labour. Hospital parking is notoriously expensive and if you go into labour during the day, parking may be limited. The last thing you want to do is have your stressed-out partner driving around looking for a parking space while you are deep-breathing on all fours in the back of the car. Local taxi companies will have taken plenty of women in labour to the hospital before, but if you're worried about your waters breaking (or they have already broken) wear lots of super-absorbent pads and put a towel on the seat.

If getting a taxi isn't an option, you can always ask a good friend or family member to drive you to hospital; that way your birth partner can sit with you in the back and help you keep focused on your breathing. People love to help out when it comes to babies, so don't be too shy to ask: you're bound to be inundated with offers.

Midwives always recommend calling the labour ward/birth centre before you go in. That way the midwife can really assess over the phone if it sounds like you should be coming into hospital. Us midwives are very good at working out how labour is progressing over the phone, and there's nothing worse than thinking you're in labour, to be sent home again as it's too soon.

Always remember the following things when you're going into hospital or the birth centre:

1 Make sure you've called and have been given the go-ahead to go in by a midwife

2 Maternity notes

3 Hospital bag for you and your baby

4 Baby car seat

5 Snack bag

6 Phone, camera and chargers

7 Fed the cat?

8 Blown out the candle you've had burning in the bathroom?

9 Turned the oven off?

10 Had a hug and kiss, this is it!

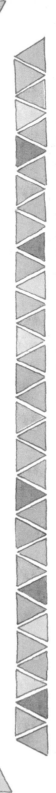

40 WEEKS

IS THIS BABY GOING
TO FALL OUT?

YOUR BABY IS ABOUT THE SIZE OF A SMALL PUMPKIN —
NEARLY 52CM (FROM HEAD TO TOE, BUT IT IS CURLED UP
INSIDE YOU) — AND WEIGHS ABOUT 3.5KG.

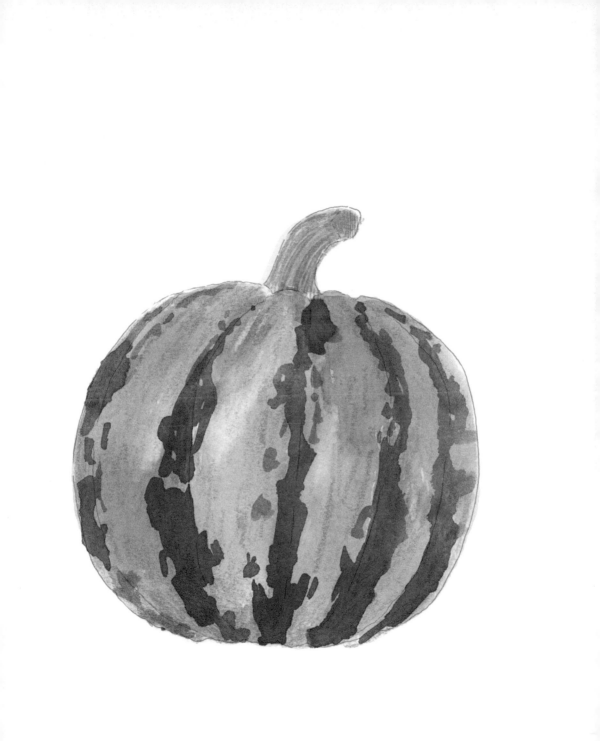

NOT FOCUSING ON YOUR DUE DATE

You will probably by now be feeling pretty pregnant, and it's fair to say by the time you reach this stage that bump is well and truly big! Everyone from the person on the checkout at your supermarket to your mum's friend from her book club will have an opinion on when this baby will arrive. (Now is a good time to start practising your 'thanks for your opinion I didn't ask for' face).

Hopefully, if you've been sensible, you haven't told the world your actual estimated due date (EDD) (see page 12). It's thought that as few as 5 per cent of babies are born on their due date, and the majority of first-time pregnancies go overdue by a week; it's no wonder women get totally fed up when there is no sign of the baby!

So here's a list of all the things you should do to keep you busy and stop your mind going crazy when you receive the tenth text of the day from yet another friend asking if you've had the baby yet? (Um, let me just check my vagina. Nope, still no baby yet).

- Don't tell the whole world when your actual due date is. Or constantly update Facebook and Twitter with '39+6. Tomorrow we will get to meet our baby'. Because, as I've just said, you probably won't have your baby on its due date unless you fall in the 5 per cent. Just add on a few days and say, 'Oh, sometime next week'.

- Meet your workmates for lunch. And remind yourself how brilliant it is that you don't have to worry about stressful deadlines and work-related politics for at least three months, a year if you're lucky.

- Read *Birth Without Fear* by Grantly Dick-Read. It's peaceful and empowering, especially if you're a little freaked out as every person you meet in the street decides to tell you their horror birth story. Yeah, thanks, really helpful.

- Put all those 'How to Be the Perfect Mother' books back on the shelf. It's not worth reading them yet, and your baby certainly hasn't read them.

Maternal instinct is an amazing thing and has guided women since the beginning of time.

- Check you've got everything in your hospital bag, and maybe even label things so your partner knows the difference between a maternity pad and a nappy. See pages 152–5.
- Go to the cinema with your partner/best mate/sister. You probably won't go again until your baby reaches his or her first birthday. And anyway, you'll be so tired you'll fall asleep halfway through and miss the big reveal. I never did see the end of *Atonement*.
- The same goes for that book sitting on your bedside table: finish it now or you'll never finish it. I started reading again when my first child was 18 months old. It was a big achievement not to be reading a five-page 'lift the flaps' book.
- Have a pedicure. Mainly because it's nice to look down at your toes after the baby has been born and not at your saggy tummy. I went for a classic red; it was bold and daring and made me feel a bit glamorous when I really felt like I had been up for three days at a warehouse rave.
- Clean your kitchen floor, on all fours. It will look shiny and clean but, more importantly, it will help get your baby into the best position for birth.
- Think about having sex with your partner. It may be the last thing you fancy doing, but it's nice to be intimate. I think 'spoons' is the only practical position to try when carrying a huge bump. But, more importantly, oxytocin (the hormone that controls your contractions) is released during sex, especially if you have an orgasm (bonus!) and semen contains prostaglandins, which can help to ripen and soften the cervix.

BIRTH STORY: THE UNPLANNED HOME BIRTH

ELLIE, SECOND BABY

Gav was spending a lot of time working in London and we took ages deliberating how we would manage if I went into labour while he was away. Friends and family had offered to be on hand to drive me to hospital, hold the fort until Gav got back, and I had a rota of potential babysitters for our son, Rufus. Nothing to worry about. That weekend, Gav was in London, and we had a couple of friends from America staying. They were new to England and we had offered to show them around Leeds. It would be nice to have company while I was heavily pregnant.

I spoke to Gav that evening, him in London, me in Leeds. 'If anything happens, keep me in the loop, Ellie.' 'Nothing is going to happen tonight, Gav, I'm 38 weeks,' said unsuspecting me.

It was a strange night; I kept waking and having pain across the top of my tummy, not like contractions. I felt worried and started to push the poor baby around with my hands, desperate to feel some movement. I slept on and off until 4 a.m., when I felt a kick... no... a pop? Had my waters broken? I stood up and there was a trickle. When I made it to the toilet there was more of a gush. I called the maternity assessment suite, who said it sounded like it could possibly be my waters and to give it an hour until I came in to be checked. Convinced my waters had broken, I called Gav: 'Get the first train back from London.' He could be back in 5 hours. Plenty of time, surely? I called my mum, and I decided I would wait for her to arrive before heading to the maternity suite.

I tried to sleep a bit more, but the adrenalin had kicked in. I got dressed and decided to make some toast and watch some telly. At 5 a.m. contractions started but I called the midwife, who said there was no rush to go in unless I thought I was in established labour. From this point on, I think I was delirious! My toast lay uneaten, the TV was never turned on. Gav kept calling telling me to use my contractions app. It was telling me that my contractions were 2 minutes apart, but I kept thinking that can't be right and clearing the whole history to start timing again! He told me to wake our visitors, but I thought it was too early in the morning and I'd be labouring for ages. I straightened my hair(?!), then felt an urge to push and went to the toilet. At this point I called my mum: 'I don't think I can wait for you (she still had an hour to go), I think I'd better call a taxi', to which she replied 'I think you'd better call an ambulance.'

178

I crouched over on the stairs on the way up to my bedroom, pain taking over my body, and called 999.

'I'm bearing down,' I told the emergency services, 'I think I'm going to have a baby!' (Who ever says 'I'm bearing down'?) She replied, 'I'm going to talk you through how to deliver your baby!' 'I'm not having it here!' I cried. She asked me if I could feel any part of the baby, I thought, hmmm can I feel the baby? Oh, I can feel the actual baby! She directed me to get sheets and towels out on the floor, which I did, but all the while I was thinking this really is stupid... then woaaaaahwhoa... it's coming.

'Arrrrrrrggghhhh!' I screamed. Yep, that woke our visitors up, for sure – and one of them rushed up the stairs, only to be greeted with 'I'm really sorry, it wasn't supposed to happen like this, but is that a head?'

'I think that's a head!' she replied. She was amazing! She took the phone from me and (while struggling to understand the Yorkshire twang) delivered Ida Rose Evelyn right there and then on my bedroom floor at 6 a.m. And wow! She was safe, she was beautiful, she was healthy, it was so peaceful. I lay with her in my arms for 8 minutes until the paramedics showed up.

I called Gav. 'I'm so sorry, I've had her!' Poor Gav, having paid £50 taxi fare to get to King's Cross, sat in the back of the taxi, gutted, the burly taxi driver comforting him.

The paramedics treated me like a queen, scurrying round my bedroom finding me bits and pieces, including some Toblerone. I was in shock! They delivered the placenta and cut the umbilical cord. Rufus woke up, and the timing could not have been more perfect. What a precious moment, walking down the stairs, Ida wrapped in a towel, to be greeted by her big brother munching his breakfast.

Off Ida and I went to hospital. She fed beautifully all the way there and I felt such a surge of love and such completeness.

Gav burst into the hospital at 9 a.m. 'We have to have a third child now so I don't miss the birth again', he said, while cradling Ida and wondering at her petite, dark features. 'Let's not talk about that right now, Gav!'

REST, EAT WELL & KEEP ACTIVE

LOOKING AFTER YOU AND BUMP

This is the perfect time to be really thinking about you and your well-being. It is a surreal time before your baby is born – a bit like going to bed as a child on Christmas Eve but waking up not knowing if Santa's been or not. Every night I would go to sleep thinking 'Is tonight the night?' only to wake up a bit more pregnant and a bit more grumpy.

You're probably feeling pretty tired most days; it's unlikely you're getting any decent sleep at the moment with all the frequent trips to the bathroom (and the constant knicker-checking: is that my show?). Having an afternoon power nap while listening to your relaxing music from your labour playlist is the perfect way to rid your mind of all those 'Have we got enough white babygrows and muslins?' thoughts. Sometimes there can be a huge feeling of pressure to have absolutely everything perfect for when the baby is born, but the reality is that perfect is unachievable and letting some things go will make life so much easier.

If you can, getting out of the house and meeting a friend for a walk can do your mind and body the world of good. Walking is a great way of getting your baby in a good position in your pelvis, and it is possible that it will bring on labour! Being upright encourages your baby to move down onto your cervix (see page 123). Then, as you walk, the rhythmic pressure of your baby's head on your cervix stimulates the release of oxytocin, which is the hormone you produce in labour and makes your uterus contract.

There are some days when you will just want to eat cheese on toast and ice cream and others when you may feel your appetite has completely gone due to your stomach being squashed by your baby. You can be healthy without having to inhale kilos of kale. As you only need 200 more calories per day in the third trimester, you don't need to eat loads more; try to eat regularly, three meals a day and, where possible, healthy snacks in between.

Tips for eating well in the lead-up to labour:

- Eat little and often to the avoid the dreaded heartburn.
- Variety is your friend! Try to include foods from the four food groups as much as possible.
- Eat foods rich in iron, like lean red meat, and leafy green vegetables such as spinach and broccoli.
- Try to have something high in fibre and wholegrain with every meal as they are filling and will keep you regular.
- Remember, it's okay to treat yourself! Naughty nibbles are fine in moderation. Sometimes chocolate is the only answer.

TO WAX OR NOT TO WAX?

And that is the question I get asked all the time as a midwife. In all honesty, it really doesn't make the slightest bit of difference to us midwives. We really don't even notice a bit of bush down there when we're about to deliver your baby. We're far more interested in seeing your baby's head!

It's also worth considering that you probably won't want to take yourself off to the beauty salon to have a wax in the first place. That area can feel really sensitive and sometimes swollen (both totally normal, by the way) at this stage in your pregnancy, so having hot wax applied down there may not be particularly appealing. Also, as with any waxing, there's the growing-back stage, which may mean ingrowing hairs and potentially spots or, even worse, a rash. If this all happens after you've given birth and you have had stitches down there, well, you can imagine how unpleasant it may become.

When I was pregnant with my first baby I was so determined to still feel like 'me' right up until the end of my pregnancy, I booked a wax on my due date, much to everyone's horror. It was pretty painful, despite having been a regular waxer previously; I guess everything down there was super-sensitive. Anyway, as much as I was convinced my baby wouldn't be 'late' he was born almost two weeks later. In that time frame my fanny wax had started to grow out and was quite itchy. I really regretted getting it done: maternity pads, bleeding and stitches were enough to contend with, let with alone a wax regrowth! It's safe to say that with my second baby, waxing was not a priority. Instead I practised my hypnobirthing techniques and had a really positive birth. And neither time did the midwife comment on my neat bikini line or overgrown bush. I guess she was more focused on delivering my baby!

Jess, mum of two

182

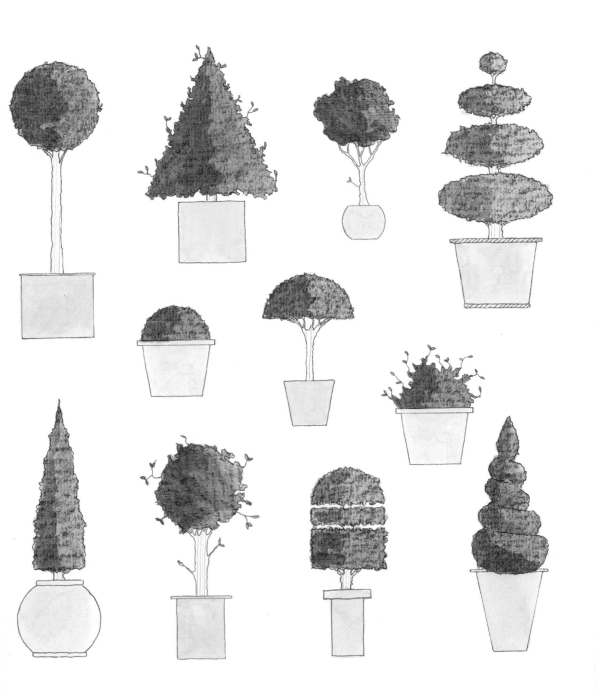

SEX: SHOULD YOU?

What a question! Sex is the reason you're pregnant in the first place, so why not think about having sex to, well, not be pregnant any more? You may be feeling too tired to even contemplate the thought of getting jiggy, not to mention the huge bump, which needs some serious logistical planning if you're going to get down to business. But if you're up for it, having sex at this stage can have the added benefit of bringing on labour.

Unless you've been told otherwise by your doctor or midwife (or if your waters have broken), sex is entirely safe at this stage of pregnancy. Whether or not you actually feel like getting in the mood with you partner is another matter. You may be feeling a bit swollen (and I don't mean your ankles) — lots of women experience swollen labia towards the end of their pregnancy due to the increased pressure from the baby on your pelvic floor. You may also be unfortunate enough to be suffering from haemorrhoids (piles). So, you may ask, why the hell would I want to have sex with all this going on?

Well, an orgasm can stimulate your uterus to start contracting. And there is strong evidence that nipple stimulation stimulates your uterus too, so a bit of foreplay could be just enough to get things going. Also, sperm contains high levels of prostaglandins that can ripen and soften your cervix.

My wife was driving me crazy at the end of the pregnancy and we tried everything to try and bring on labour, but when it came to sex I was hesitant. I was a bit grossed out by the idea and I was pretty sure I was going to take the little one's eye out with my manhood, but I was assured that no man is that well endowed, so we did it. However, our son was born nine days later after a pretty arduous induction. My wife likes to think he gets his stubborn tendencies from me.

Sam, father of one

IS THIS LABOUR? SIGNS THAT THIS COULD BE IT!

As with anything pregnancy- and birth-related, everyone is different, so just because your sister had a show and went into labour that day it doesn't mean the same will happen to you. Just for the record, I had a show with my first baby on my due date. Bingo, I thought, how super-efficient my body is! I went into labour five days later. And even with my knowledge and expertise as a midwife, by this stage, I, too, had become obsessed with any body fluid in my knickers every time I went to the loo. So don't worry if you are checking your discharge every hour, you're not alone! You may experience:

- A bloody show (mucus including either brown old blood or fresh blood).
- Your waters might go – sometimes this can be a slow trickle.
- Diarrhoea and/or feeling nauseous.
- Dull lower backache that may require paracetamol to 'take the edge off it'.
- Achy tops of the thighs.
- Irregular stomach cramps that can often feel like period pains.
- A sensation of not quite feeling right.

> I felt like I do just before I get my period when I went into labour, really achy around my groin and cervix. All I wanted to do was curl up on the sofa with a hot water bottle. Paracetamol helped too.
> *Kirsty, mum of one*

The most important thing to remember, as I've mentioned before (see page 124), is to take it slowly. These signs that you might be going into labour can tease you for a few days before real labour starts (especially if this is your first baby). Rest up and don't announce it to the world – it might be a false alarm.

TOP TIPS - CHECKLIST

Waiting for a baby to be born is possibly the most exciting, nerve-racking but mind-boggling thing you will experience. You know that your baby will be here one way or another but you just can't believe it will ever happen. This baby, whom you haven't even met and have no idea what he or she looks like, will be in your arms sometime during the next two weeks. To keep your mind sane and your hands busy, here are some ideas for things to be doing. (Note: I did all of these with every pregnancy, so can confidently vouch that they really helped me when my phone pinged for the 99th time that day with another friend or relative asking 'any signs?'

- Ironing – never before had I ever ironed so much, but I managed to iron everything I could get my hands on: white babygrows, duvet covers, tea towels, you name it, it was ironed and folded into neat little piles. Plus standing is a great way to keep that baby in a good position in your pelvis (see UFO, page 123).
- Do an online shop – get some really delicious 'treat' foods in: ice cream, your favourite chocolate, perhaps those posh ready-meals. The likelihood is you'll be really knackered come 8 p.m. and cooking can seem like such a chore, plus you can freeze it if you don't end up eating it now and save it for after the baby is born.
- Nappy/baby wipe/muslin check – buy these in bulk with your online shop so you don't run out in the first month. Supermarkets often have '3 for 2' offers on, so take advantage.
- Same goes for household essentials – loo roll, milk, dishwasher tablets. Your partner will not want to 'pop' out to the shops when your baby is three days old because you've run out of loo roll, trust me.
- Finish watching that box set – I was heavily engrossed in a real-life crime story that I had to finish before the twins arrived. How could I possibly labour not knowing whodunnit?

- Make up the Moses basket/crib – this is a pretty special moment, no matter what number baby it is and got me feeling super-emotional every time I did it. Nothing says 'we're ready to meet you, baby' than a white fitted sheet, folded blanket and soft rabbit placed perfectly in the crib. Sob!
- Nap! Every afternoon, on the sofa or in bed; it's really important you rest your body before you go into labour. A well-rested mind and body is essential for feeling calm and focused. You can do this!
- If this isn't your first baby, then ask friends if they can take your older child off your hands for an afternoon. It will give you a breather and allow your child (or children) to enjoy playing at someone else's house.

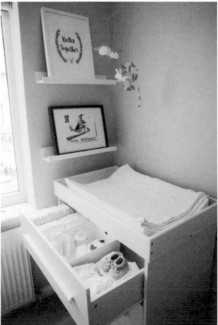

- There are some lovely illustrated books for children about to become a big brother/sister – this can really help them to understand the changes that are going to happen, why Mummy might be very tired and why Grandma or Grandpa might be collecting them from nursery on several occasions.
- Give your child realistic expectations of a newborn baby in the house – we told our daughters that tiny babies were boring, cried and slept lots. That way they didn't feel disappointed when their three-day-old twin baby sisters didn't want to play tea parties.

BIRTH STORY: A FIRST-TIME BIRTH WITH AN EPIDURAL

HELEN, FOUNDER OF LIONHEART MAGAZINE, FIRST BABY

Like most expectant mothers, I didn't know exactly how the process would go, but I was ready. I'd done the classes, eaten the cake and stretched like a pregnant yoga cat. A day over your due date is fine, so is a week. Less so when 13 days pass and nothing happens. Needles stuck in me. Raspberry-leaf tea with pineapple chasers, fire curry for starters. Stretch and sweep times three. 'They do tend to come when they're ready,' on repeat. Our induction was booked for day 14 but the poppet made her first gentle movements to leave her haven on day 13. It started with a gentle jolt at 5 a.m. It was the tightening combined with twinges that I had been waiting for.

I had opted for a home birth. We had everything ready: pool, towels, chocolate, tea and biscuits for the midwives, candles and flowers on the mantelpiece. We went for coffee and wandered around. All the while, my contractions were 9–10 minutes apart. By the evening, they were 5 minutes apart, so I rang the hospital. Not strong enough or regular enough. 'Get some rest,' said the voice at the end of the phone.

The midwife popped in at 11 a.m. the next morning. 'You're 3cm.' How could this be after 30 hours? She continued: 'I think something is stopping your progress. You should go to the hospital, just to check everything's okay.'

We were taken through to the midwife-led unit, a luxurious hotel of birthing, complete with pools, beds, floor pillows, birth balls, private bathrooms and fairy lights. I was told the pool is a source of pain relief, as was the gas and air, so it was best to hold out as long as possible to use both of them. We were shown to our room. I stripped off and bounced on the birth ball, clinging to Charlie's belt. Very quickly an imprint of the buckle formed on my forehead – nice. Time melted and the world became deep and wide (interesting in retrospect!).

God, I didn't have a care. Just this baby, just this intense, empowering experience. My entire body was being taken over with its own innate superpowers. I really was off and away, smiling from under a canopy of hormones and focus. The midwife could have told me that Ryan Gosling was in my birth pool and I would have simply smiled, nodded, closed my eyes and furrowed my brow. I think it was the pregnancy yoga that zoned me.

Who knows – maybe some fairy godmother made a trip to see me. Anyway, I was finally allowed in the pool – hurrah! – at 5cm.

Dear Pool, I loved you so. However, after an hour, my baby did not like it in there and the squirrel's heart rate zoomed up. I had to get out of the watery haven and lie on the bed to have my waters broken. The breaking signified change. Post-break my hands tingled, I felt dehydrated, exhausted and actual pain hit me for the first time. What's more, I hadn't dilated any further – the midwife said. In actual fact, I'd gone down to 4cm. I went heavy on the gas and air. My smug little Zen space had officially exploded.

After 4 hours our midwife told me that I had not progressed at all. I have no words to express how this felt. It had been 40-plus hours since that first contraction. The midwife suggested we go downstairs to The Drip. Or we could continue to wait, but she was concerned I was shattered, which I was. Previously, 'downstairs' symbolised all that I didn't desire for my baby's birth, but at this point it became exactly what I needed. The words tumbled out of my mouth: 'Please can I have an epidural?' Bleugh. The midwife replied that with the drip speeding up contractions, it would be wise and I would need my energy for pushing. Gosh.

The lights dimmed. Bill Callahan playing softly, a view of the city's lights. Charlie snoozing on the floor and the sweet, regular sound of our baby's heartbeat. This was a different place, one of calm and a gathering of thoughts. This was the epidural I thought I would never have. It pulled me back to where I needed to be. It gave me rest, peace and that wonderful focus back again.

After a few hours of dozing and chatting I was 10cm and ready to push. I'd made sure to stop the epidural switch earlier to feel as much as I could. I was soon instructed to puuuush with all my might, taking short breaks to take in more air. I pushed and imagined holding my baby in my arms. I could feel the baby coming. I absolutely loved this very active part.

It took just 10 minutes for this beautiful, crying, wriggling, eyes-wide-awake baby to emerge. The midwife unwrapped the cord around the baby's neck and handed our baby to me, whereupon my body absolutely flooded me with hormones and love.

Annoyingly, I had quite a lot of blood loss and a couple of other complications post-birth, but the medical staff were fantastic, as was Charlie. We had a few rounds of tea and biscuits, Alba had some more colostrum, I had a blood transfusion, Charlie gave us an inflatable tiger balloon and everything felt rosy. We were floating on a cloud.

41 WEEKS

WILL I BE PREGNANT FOR EVER?!

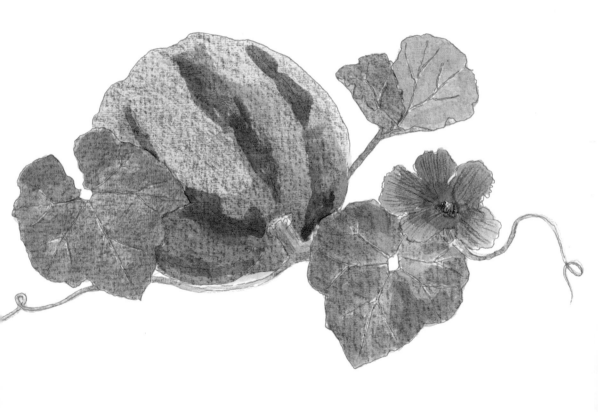

PREPARING FOR BEING INDUCED

As a midwife I have seen hundreds of births and many of those have been in the form of an induction. This section of the book is to help you if you're being induced. It's not to scare you, or give you false expectations.

Try to remember that not every induction is the same and what might work for one person might not work for someone else. Be open-minded, positive and remain focused. As always, speak to your midwife if you have any further questions – they will be more than happy to answer them.

'Induction' means to start your labour artificially, either with synthetic hormones administered into your body or by having your waters broken (artificial rupture of membranes). You will be offered an induction if the risk of prolonging your pregnancy is more serious than the risk of your baby being born sooner. You may have been advised that induction is the safest option for you and your baby if:

- You are diabetic.
- You have pre-eclampsia.
- The fluid around your baby is too much (polyhydramnios) or too little (oligohydramnios).
- Your placenta is not working effectively.
- Your baby is not growing at a normal rate.
- Your waters have broken but labour has not started naturally within 24–48 hours.
- You are 'overdue'.

Why you are being induced will decide where you will be induced. For example, if you're overdue but 'low-risk' you will most likely be induced on an antenatal ward. This ward usually consists of a four-bedded bay (with curtains around you for privacy) with other women who may also be being induced or are being kept in for observation. It's a good idea to take a pillow with you, some earplugs and eye mask, as induction may take a day or two before anything actually happens and hospital wards are noisy at night. You want to get as much sleep as possible, when you can, so you're not too tired when the real work starts!

If you're being induced for a medical reason and are being considered 'high-risk' you will most likely be induced on the labour ward. Depending on the hospital you may have a shared bay or a single room.

HOW IS INDUCTION CARRIED OUT?

Prostaglandins
Prostaglandin is a hormone-like substance that causes your cervix to ripen, and which may stimulate contractions. Your midwife will insert a tablet, pessary or gel containing prostaglandin into your vagina. The slow-release pessary looks a bit like a small tampon. While you wait for prostaglandins to work you can usually go for a walk. You may be able to go home for up to six hours or until your contractions start. How you are given prostaglandin depends on whether this is your first or second baby. If this is your first baby, you may need a second dose of a tablet or gel after six hours.

Artificial rupture of membranes (ARM)
Artificially rupturing the membranes, also called breaking the waters, isn't recommended as a first method of induction unless vaginal prostaglandins can't be used. However, some doctors or midwives may use ARM as part of the induction process or to speed up your labour if it's not progressing. Your

midwife or doctor makes a small break in the membranes around your baby with a long, thin probe (amnihook).

An ARM often works when the cervix feels soft and ready for labour to start. It can be quite uncomfortable, so you may be offered gas and air to help you to cope. ARM doesn't always get labour started, and once your waters have been broken, your baby could be at risk of infection. That's why it's no longer recommended as a method of induction on its own and is best used after labour has started.

Syntocinon

Syntocinon is a synthetic form of the hormone oxytocin, which makes you contract. You will only be offered it if a membrane sweep or prostaglandin hasn't started your labour, or if your contractions aren't effective. Your waters have to be broken before you can be given Syntocinon.

You'll have Syntocinon through an intravenous drip, allowing the hormone to go straight into your bloodstream through a tiny tube inserted into a vein in your arm. Once your contractions have begun, the rate of the drip can be adjusted. This allows contractions to happen often enough to make your cervix dilate, without becoming too powerful.

Syntocinon is started at a very low dose and increased gradually to prevent it from stimulating your uterus or causing stress to your baby. Syntocinon can cause strong contractions and put your baby under stress, so you will need to be monitored continuously. The contractions brought on by Syntocinon may be more painful than natural ones, so you may choose to have an epidural for pain relief.

Other things to remember

Some hospitals may have the option of using a telemetry monitoring (wireless) so you can walk around and not be confined to the bed. Ask for the use of mats, balls, a birthing stool, and remember you DO NOT HAVE TO LIE ON THE BED. Not every induction means the use of Syntocinon, but you may want to consider trying the drip without an epidural to give your baby a good chance of getting into a better position for birth (epidurals increase the rate of having an instrumental delivery, see page 143).

Make sure you discuss each stage of your induction with you midwife/doctor to make sure you and your birth partner understand all options and that you can make an informed choice.

A MEMBRANE SWEEP

It may sound horrifying, but a sweep is actually fairly simple. A membrane sweep is when a midwife sweeps their finger around the opening of your cervix, which can help labour to start. Your midwife may offer you a sweep if you are full-term and waiting for labour to start or you may choose to wait. They'll suggest a sweep at your 40-week appointment if this is your first baby or at your 41-week appointment if you've had a baby before.

During a sweep, your midwife carefully separates the membranes that surround your baby from your cervix to stimulate the production of prostaglandin (this isn't breaking your waters). If your cervix is not dilated enough to do a sweep, they may stretch or massage your cervix instead. You may be offered two or three membrane sweeps. It can be uncomfortable if your cervix is difficult to reach, and you may need to have several membrane sweeps before labour starts. If your midwife has been successful with the sweep, and your cervix is forward enough for them to reach it, they should be able to tell you how soft and open it is. This may give you (although not always) a bit of an indication of how close or ready you are to going into labour. Some women experience a bit of light bleeding after a sweep, which is normal. But if you're at all worried about anything speak to your midwife.

> It felt similar to a smear but nowhere near as uncomfortable. It was over fairly quickly. I thought about something else and then it was done. Plus, by the time you are begging for your midwife to stick her fingered, covered gloves up your bits you're ready for anything.
>
> *Zoe, mum of two*

> My midwife looked a bit red in the face trying to find my cervix but eventually she got it. Deep-breathing techniques helped me stay calm.
>
> *Anna, mum of one*

NATURAL WAYS TO INDUCE LABOUR

Let me start by saying that there really is no 'magic button' to make that baby come out! Lots of natural induction methods concentrate on relaxing and restoring the mum-to-be, and in turn helping her to let go of any tension that might be causing her body to hold on. Our busy lifestyles and constant juggling of work and family often leaves us with very high levels of adrenalin, a hormone that does not do us any favours in the birthing room, and actually inhibits the production of oxytocin – our lovely birth hormone! So, when trying natural induction methods, focus on things that make you feel calm, happy and relaxed. Whatever you decide to do, do your research first, and if using a therapist, make sure they are properly qualified.

- Massage, reflexology and acupuncture all work in this way, while having the added benefit of working on certain points that are believed to stimulate the body to get ready for labour (see page 67 for some massage tips).
- Nipple stimulation also produces oxytocin.
- Lots of women swear by eating dates (six dates a day in the last four weeks of pregnancy!), pineapple, hot curries and evening primrose oil (orally or internally, this imitates prostaglandin and helps ripen the cervix). I often hear of women using castor oil to bring on contractions, but I'm not a big fan of this because castor oil can cause diarrhoea and vomiting. Who wants to deal with more of that than they need to in labour?
- I'm a big fan of using the stairs to get labour going. Walking up and down the stairs sideways increases the opening of the pelvis, allowing the baby to drop down and put more pressure on the cervix.
- Lastly one of my favourite pieces of advice I was given, and one that definitely worked for me, was from my own midwife, who told me at 41 weeks to 'go home, have a glass of fizz and a bubble bath, and then get your leg over'. We did, and it worked!

BIRTH STORY: INDUCTION

KATE, SECOND BABY

I was determined to have a relaxed home birth. I borrowed a pool, collected more old towels and bedding than I knew what to do with, and readied an army of babysitters to look after Albert, my first son. Except William had other plans. Due date came and went, no sign. Daily sweeps told me that I was 3cm dilated with a 'favourable' cervix, but it seemed that no amount of bouncing on a ball, long walks or vacuuming the stairs was going to move him along. I was due to be booked in for an induction, but decided, after a chat with my midwives, to leave him for a few more days to see if he fancied vacating of his own accord. Still nothing, and the chances of my home birth disappeared. I trudged into the hospital, only to be told that although, yes, I was still 3–4cm dilated, and yes, my waters should just be broken so that we could get on with it, sadly, they were extremely busy and had no staff or space. I reacted in the way that any massively overdue, hormonal woman would do and cried, huffed and puffed at my husband, then settled down to watch *Homes Under the Hammer* on the iPad.

I hadn't, however, banked on the appearance of my midwife, Vanessa, at 10.30 p.m. on a Friday night. She breezed into the ward, rolled up her sleeves, and very kindly instructed me that we were 'going to meet this baby. Tonight.' She found a delivery suite, settled us in, and promptly broke my waters. She found a mat and a blanket for my husband and told him to have a nap because he 'wasn't going to be much use yet' and left me to get on with it. Brilliant.

The room was lovely and calm. There was a docking station, so I left my iPod on shuffle. (The fear that the next song could be Wham kept me going, to be honest.) My contractions started pretty immediately after my waters went and became regular quickly. I was on my feet and moving around the room, stopping to lean on furniture and hum when the contractions came. After around 90 minutes, the contractions were getting much stronger, and had moved downwards into my lower back. Humming had turned more into growling and I wasn't so much leaning on the furniture as clinging to it at this point. Vanessa asked how I was doing. 'I think I need to push,' I said, surprising both of us. 'Hmm, you'd better take your pants off, then,' came the reply. By this time, I was scorching hot, so I stripped off every last stitch. Amazing what those hormones do to you. My husband made himself useful with cool flannels and encouraging words, and I was examined – I was 8.5 centimetres, but still had work to do before I could push.

Vanessa advised me to try lying on my side on a mat on the floor. I was dubious at first – gravity didn't seem to be on my side – but that shows what I know. Contractions started coming along thick and fast, and I had some gas and air to take the edge off. I'm not entirely sure that the gas had much effect, but the mouthpiece and regularity of using it was a useful distraction from pain and helped me to focus on breathing. What felt like two minutes later (but was actually about 40) the urge to push returned. This time I got the green light and a delighted voice from the other end told me 'I can see the head!' We had already ascertained that he was a big baby, so hurrying this next part could have been disastrous. I followed Vanessa's every instruction about pushing, stopping, puffing – to be honest, if she'd told me to stand up and do the Macarena I would have – and a few minutes later William's head emerged. A couple more pushes and the rest of him followed, all 9lbs 5oz of him, with not a single tear, graze or stitch. There was a calm sense of amazement in the room afterwards – I was staggered that my body had done what it needed to so efficiently after a slow start – and we were all dazzled by this enormous (and beautiful!) baby.

Although I was in a busy hospital, it felt like there was only me, my husband and Vanessa in the world, and then William too! It was calm, I was calm, and William's welcome into the world was calm and overwhelmingly happy. The whole process took three hours from start to finish, and I was home and introducing William to his big brother two hours later. If you find yourself having an induction or hospital delivery that you didn't hope for, don't despair!

DECIDING TO BE INDUCED OR TO WAIT? WHAT'S SAFE?

You've tidied the house from top to bottom, your kitchen floor is squeaky clean (see page 177), the bag is packed, the Moses basket is ready, you've gyrated on your birth ball, hell you've even tweaked your nipples AND done the unthinkable – had sex… but still no baby. You're probably feeling a bit fed up, and remembering that only around 5 per cent of babies are born on their due date isn't making you feel better. What next?

Your midwife will have offered you one (or more) sweeps and you may decide to try some alternative therapies to get things going. Most hospitals follow the national guidelines, which recommend offering induction when you're 41 weeks pregnant. This is based on evidence that babies are healthier at birth and are more likely to be born safe and well when hospitals induce labour at, or beyond, 41 weeks. You could also request a 'post-dates' scan to check on your baby's well-being, including the functioning of the amniotic fluid and the placenta. But, like anything, a scan isn't always going to be 100 per cent accurate and could be interpreted in different ways. The risk of fetal distress and stillbirth is increased after 42 weeks, particularly for women expecting their first baby. However, even though the rate increases, having a baby who is stillborn between 39–42 weeks is still rare. The stillbirth rate is less than one in 1,000 babies at 39–40 weeks, increasing to around one in 1,000 at 41 weeks, two in 1,000 at 42 weeks and three in 1,000 babies at 43 weeks. It may be difficult to absorb those statistics, especially when you're heavily pregnant and feeling hormonal, but it's important to understand the risk, although very small, before you make an informed decision about being induced or waiting a bit longer. Remember that you should feel supported by your midwife and obstetrician whatever you decide.

RECAP ON HYPNOBIRTHING

HOLLIE DE CRUZ, LONDON HYPNOBIRTHING AND @THEYESMUMMUM

So you're 41 weeks' pregnant and there's no sign of your baby. With external pressures about induction and an eagerness to meet your baby, it's easy to see why you might be feeling stressed and fed up at this point, so let's recap on why it's actually all good! Feeling anxious is the last thing you need right now. When we feel this way, we produce cortisol and adrenalin – our stressor hormones and the very things that prevent us from going into labour – so it's really important that we short-circuit this response by replacing them with happy hormones. Remember the endorphins and oxytocin we love in hypnobirthing? It's time to bring out those bad boys.

I know it's easier said than done when you're lugging around a full-term human being, but it's what you need to do to bring them earthside. Disconnect from the outside world so that you can tune in to your baby and yourself. Use positive affirmations to remind yourself that it's all as it should be – things like 'my baby will arrive when the time is right' or 'my baby knows how and when to be born'. And tell your baby that it's safe too, that you're excited to meet him or her and that you're ready. Nurture yourself with warm baths, a massage and quiet, private space. Recap on your breathing techniques, especially if you're experiencing Braxton Hicks.

And remember that your baby is not late. Anything between 37–42 weeks is completely normal for your baby to be born, so trust the process. Plan something lovely for yourself each day and indulge in this sacred time, where you and your baby are one for the last time. Rest when you are tired, and thank your body for the beautiful journey it's been on. Visualise your calm, empowering birth experience; visualise your body working exactly as it's meant to – powerfully, comfortably and efficiently; visualise holding your baby in your arms. It is all coming to you, and you can do it.

GOING 'OVERDUE'

CLEMMIE TELFORD, @CLEMMIE_TELFORD

Babies don't have a diary in the womb. Which means they turn up when they are ready. Sometimes this can be a bit 'later' than you had hoped. This is perfectly normal. But, as with everything pregnancy-related, it can make you go a bit loopy.

I went 'over' with both my boys. And this is how I behaved:

- Felt angry towards friends for giving birth when they should have known it was my turn.
- Cried hysterically with jealousy of the above.
- Thought/felt as if I might actually stay pregnant for ever.
- Searched on the Internet for: 'longest pregnancy in history.'
- Hated everyone who told me to have curry and pineapple.
- While scoffing both in vast quantities anyway.
- Attempted the unthinkable: had sex.
- Discussed concerns about hubby's willy potentially poking baby's head.
- Pleaded with my body to feel pain. When else in life are you desperate to feel an agonising cramp?
- Studied my discharge extensively.
- Discussed my discharge extensively.
- Thought every poo was a 'sign'.
- Thought every fart was a 'sign'.
- Ate all the snacks from my birth bag.
- Twice.
- Spent over £100 on alternative therapy trying to get baby out.
- Cursed anyone who told me their baby was early, for 'bragging'.
- Sulked.
- Attempted 'self-examination' to determine possible dilation. Failed.
- Swore that 'this child takes after its father.' I'm always punctual.

- Swayed back and forth between thinking I desperately wanted an induction NOW, to thinking I'd definitely decline an induction.
- Asked my poor mum, who'd come to take care of me, to go elsewhere because I couldn't stand the pressure of her being in the house.
- Began every day optimistically thinking that 'today is the day'. Only to get to 7 p.m. feeling miserable that yet again it wasn't.
- Cried.
- Went over and over and over and over the plans for what would happen to my first boy when I did eventually go into labour.
- Said things like 'It'd be awful if it came during that rugby match/dinner party' while deep down thinking it'd be excellent if it came any time at all.
- Sulked.
- Felt more like a failure with every passing day.
- Questioned every baby name we had on our shortlist.
- Cried.
- Gave up wearing anything but joggers. Those maternity clothes were taunting me.
- Had evil thoughts about everybody who texted saying 'any news??' YOU'LL KNOW WHEN THE BABY IS HERE, YOU NOSEY PARKER.
- Felt like a mug for all those weeks of counting down to a now-irrelevant date.
- Realised I am definitely a control freak.
- And then eventually had a baby and instantly forgot about all the above.

AND THEN WE WERE A FAMILY

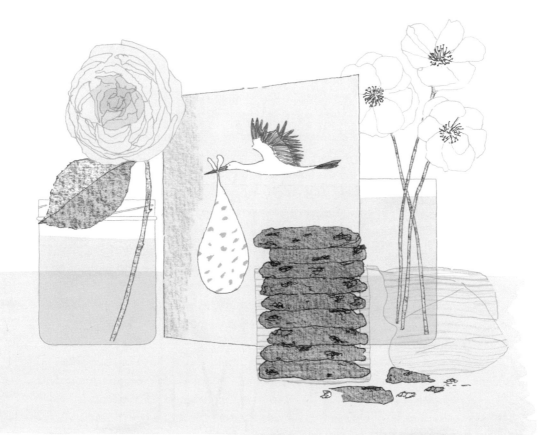

COPING IN THOSE EARLY DAYS

ANNA WHITEHOUSE, @MOTHER_PUKKA

I don't want to gild the lily here because we all know birth nips a bit, and equally adjusting to those first few weeks takes some serious boobs/balls. But batten down the hatches and you might make it through with only a mid-level eye twitch with all relationships vaguely intact.

1 Don't do anything. It sounds simple, almost relaxing. But your instinct is to join the world and show people you are on this, that you have not changed. You have changed. Your fanny and stomach have changed, your sleep has changed and you've made a human. That's some big shit right there. Let all that sink in and ask friends and family to make that quinoa beetroot cake you feel might make everything okay.

2 Stack up the snacks. The most annoying thing for everyone involved is those moments of 'darling, could you just pass me… [insert 'my phone/ biscuit/essential life item']. Find a table and treat it like your pencil case at the start of a new school term, when you made sure you had all the right stuff. This is no different, stack that snack station up and get all the reading material you need. Feeding babies is really boring; if you can master the feeding/scrolling Instagram set-up, you are winning.

3 Tell mates if you are not okay. There's nothing more uniting than adversity. I don't like to see my mates in a pickle, but I love to have the opportunity of showing the love. That love can come in a hug, home-made shepherd's pie or just a grotty Tinder story from 'the other world'. Just because you have a mate who doesn't have kids, doesn't mean she won't get it.

4 Let everyone do everything. Again sounds simple, almost relaxing. But the sooner you can let go of trying to do everything perfectly your way, the sooner you'll understand this whole keeping-humans-alive thing is a massive group task. If you have a mate who will hold the baby when you need a wee, then you are golden.

PARTNER'S PERSPECTIVE

SIMON HOOPER, @FATHER_OF_DAUGHTERS

Those first weeks of being a family can be challenging, especially the first time around. This is when dads need to step up and earn their keep.

My role during those first weeks when I was on paternity leave was a combination of chef, PA, security and logistics manager – all rolled into one. I made sure that everything ran smoothly while minimising the amount of 'stuff' that could cause my other half to get stressed out (and, as you well know, a calm relaxed woman equals a calm relaxed house and an easier life for you!) Here's some tips on things to stay on top of:

- Cleaning: nesting women are mental. They like everything sparkling, so avoid arguments and do your best with the antibacterial spray. It may not be up to her standards, but at least you're making an effort.
- Bed rest: your partner should be having a couple of days in bed when you get home. Make sure you're there to get things, sign for deliveries and generally be a dogsbody, so she doesn't have to be up and about.
- Sleep: when the baby is asleep, you should encourage your partner to be as well. Sleep is a precious commodity in those early weeks, so enforce it when you can (for both her and your own sanity).
- Food: make sure your partner eats regularly. She'll likely only want small nibbles but she'll need them on a fairly frequent basis, so make sure you've got the food in the house she likes/wants/needs.
- Visitors: you've got to control the flow of people and make sure they don't outstay their welcome – no visitors outside of direct family in the first two days is a good rule to start with.
- Positive messaging: your partner is going to be on a bit of an emotional seesaw. Tell her positive things about how she's doing. Be calm, be kind and be patient. It WILL make a difference.

BREASTFEEDING: SUPPORT NETWORKS

Sometimes the most natural of things are the most difficult. With all the planning and preparing in the world (see pages 110–11) breastfeeding can, for some, be a real struggle. I struggled with each of my four babies when it came to feeding and all for different reasons. And I'm a midwife! It's definitely not automatically easier for the 'experts'.

It can, at times, feel like the 'blind leading the blind' – neither of you have done it before and it can take lots and lots of practice before you've got it right. That may be within the first week, or longer, it doesn't matter either way. What matters is that you ask for help when you're struggling.

ALISON, MUM OF ONE

I breastfed my daughter, Grace, for six months and to start with, it was incredibly difficult. All of the advice and 'practice' we'd had in our NCT classes suddenly felt a million miles away from the reality of having a newborn trying to latch on to my breast! It felt a bit like having this incredibly complex puzzle to solve – putting the bits in exactly the right way and order, for it to work. And on next to no sleep and with crazy hormones buzzing around my body. It's fair to say, it was tough!

I struggled for the first few days and the midwives in the maternity ward were great at giving me tips when I asked for help. However, remembering the tips when it was feeding time was another challenge! And then, once we were doing it correctly, and Grace was feeding properly, THE PAIN! Oh, it makes my eyes water just thinking about it. Thankfully this didn't last long, and we soon got into a rhythm of feeding every three hours or so. My husband, Mark, and my mum were usually on hand to make sure I had water, nipple cream, a snack, the TV remote and muslins nearby because in the early days, feeding could take up to an hour.

But I'm so glad we persevered. It got loads easier and soon I was whacking Grace on my boob for a feed without a care in the world. I was very self-conscious about feeding in public, which, looking back, is such a shame that society made me feel like this. I tended to find feeding rooms in shopping centres or scurry home to feed her, rather than do it in a café or restaurant. It was an extra pressure I didn't actually need.

When Grace got to six months and we started weaning her on to solids, as it felt, for us, like the right time to stop breastfeeding. I remember having a desire to 'get my boobs back' after feeling like they weren't really 'mine' for six months. If I had a second, I might try to breastfeed for longer.

- Don't be disheartened if you find breastfeeding tough to start with. I don't know anyone who finds it easy.
- Ask for help. There are breastfeeding clinics and support groups who are there to give advice and show you what to do (see page 220 for more info).
- Don't hide away like I did! There's nothing embarrassing about breastfeeding and if anyone gives you a look, just ignore them.
- Stop when it feels right for you. Don't pay attention to any pressure to breastfeed for longer, or shorter, than you want to. You know what's best for you and your child.

COPING WITH VISITORS

Having a baby is huge, joyous occasion that brings everyone together to celebrate this brand-new human being, not to mention you and your partner becoming parents. But with all their good intentions, visitors are exhausting for any new parent. So what is the right thing to do when friends and family are desperate to come and see you and your new baby? You will no doubt be in your PJs resting in bed most days (which is exactly what you should be doing) and welcoming guests when you haven't even opened the curtains and the dirty plates from three days ago are still in the kitchen can all seem too much to cope with. But given clear messages prior to the doorbell ringing, visitors can be an amazing asset to exhausted, sleep-deprived parents.

- Food. A simple store-cupboard staple such as biscuits and a pint of milk are far more essential than new-baby presents. I still remember the lasagne brought by a neighbour when the twins were born. I cried, it was so kind.
- Set a time limit. One person's too-long is another person's warm-up. But when it comes to visitors, limit it to 45 minutes to one hour maximum. Your energy is limited and there's a hit-by-a-bus vibe in the air for a good couple of weeks after birth.
- Ask for help. Depending on the closeness of the friendship, 'helpful' can range from rinsing out your own tea cups to putting out the rubbish. Suggest specific tasks rather than staring hopefully at the dishwasher. Ask someone to take the baby for a walk so you can go to bed or have a long bath. Those small luxuries are few and far between in the beginning.

Try to spend as much time in bed nuzzling your newborn as possible. When I had the twins I didn't leave the bedroom for the first week, AND IT WAS BLISS. Those early days are so precious, but lots of new mums are desperate to go out and try the new pram/sling. There will be plenty of time to do that. Enjoy this time.

DRESSING YOUR POST-BABY BODY

ZOE DE PASS, DRESS LIKE A MUM

After birth your body will change and will keep changing for some time while it recovers from pregnancy. It is important not to put any pressure on yourself to fit straight back into your pre-pregnancy clothes – you can get there and there is no hurry.

- Post-labour you will be feeling a bit fragile, so always opt for comfy, cosy, soft clothes. Invest in some tracksuit bottoms you love (chances are you will want to wear these a lot), look for stretchy, soft waistbands and make sure they are washable: babies can be messy. Get some soft T-shirts and vests that can be worn under things.
- If you invested in maternity clothes while you were pregnant, then these will be good to keep wearing post-labour as they will now fit on the looser side and feel comfortable, which ultimately is the most important thing. Look for clothes that you can breastfeed in and that are practical for when you are playing with the kids.
- Loose shirts and shirt dresses can be good; most probably your breasts will have got a lot bigger and your stomach needs time to recover from growing a human. These can be worn over your maternity jeans, leggings, shorts or skirts and you can wear things under and on top of them too.
- Jumpsuits can be great and are comfortable (avoid ones with waistbands, especially if you have had a C-section), as they are an easy, quick outfit-in-one. Dungarees are good, too, as they are flattering on the tummy and breasts and are perfect for breastfeeding.
- The key is to feel comfortable and happy. Chances are people will be more interested in looking at your new baby than you, so don't worry.

EAT, SLEEP, POO, REPEAT

If there's one true fact about having a newborn baby in your life, it's that your sleep patterns are about to become massively altered. Those carefree nights of eight hours' sleep will be a distant memory, as your baby will keep you busy with what will seem like endless feeding, winding and changing. It's incredible that something so small can demand so much from you at hours you haven't seen since your partying days.

There is no easy way of getting used to the broken sleep – four children later I'm still adjusting – but with some realistic expectations and tips here and there you may find it a tiny bit easier.

WHAT TO EXPECT

Babies have a high biological need to eat regularly; their tiny tummies start off only the size of a cherry, so they empty quickly and they need to be re-filled again.

You may also wonder how your baby can sleep for long periods during the day but as soon as night comes he or she wants to feed like a mad thing. Your oxytocin and prolactin levels are elevated at night, which means you produce more milk, which in turn encourages your baby to feed more frequently. Also, the sleep hormone melatonin isn't fully produced by babies until at least 9 to 12 weeks (when the pineal gland matures). Until then, breastfed babies receive melatonin from breast milk. The main thing you'll notice is that your baby will not know the difference between day and night.

Although it may be hard, it's a good idea if you can try to adapt your sleeping patterns to your baby's. While this may be easier said than done, having an afternoon nap every day when your baby sleeps will give you and your body a little boost for getting through the next evening. This is why it's a good idea not to book in any visitors during this time. Sleep is key for surviving these early days. Sleep deprivation can push you to the lowest of lows, so sleep whenever you can and rope in a relative or friend so you can sneak off for a nap. And remember; it won't be like this for ever!

Don't get too caught up in those baby-routine books. You have to remember that your baby hasn't read them, so don't put too much pressure on the situation by trying to enforce some sort of routine. Babies are supposed to wake every two to three hours at night; it's normal for their development. Even if your NCT friend's baby is sleeping through, every baby is different.

Poo: what goes in must come out! If babies eat roughly every two to three hours then they will need to empty their tiny tummies regularly to make space for their next feed. Never underestimate how many nappies you will go through: on average, a breastfed baby will poo six times a day. Their poo will start off as a dark, black tar-like substance called meconium, then change to green and by day five or six it should be a yellowish mustard colour and very runny.

MILESTONES FOR MUMS

We've all heard of milestones for your baby – first smile, first time he slept through the night – but what about you? My God, you've achieved so much already, you need a serious fist-pump to say 'you've done it'.

- The first poo (and I don't mean your baby's) – the thought is always worse than the actual motion. Don't hold on to it either – better out than in!
- And what about dealing with the first 'poo-nami' – sometimes chucking away the baby vest is the only course of action.
- Leaving the house with clean hair – that bottle of dry shampoo won't last for ever and there's nothing like the feeling of freshly washed hair.
- First day you go it alone – your partner has gone back to work and you've kept a small human alive all day and survived on chocolate biscuits and daytime TV. You're amazing!
- First trip out with your baby – it took you two hours to actually leave the house and you're only walking to your local shops, but how many spare changes of clothes and nappies does one tiny human need? (See point 2.)
- Getting into your non-maternity jeans – you may not be able to do them up or even contemplate eating in them but they're on. Just.
- Successfully folding and collapsing the pram alone – without trapping your fingers in the process or dropping the baby. Winning at life.
- First time you breastfeed in front of your father-in-law – it gets all a bit hot and sweaty as you casually try to hide under a massive muslin and pray your baby stays latched on for once. Cue nipple exposure.
- First night out without your baby – even though you and your partner are either too sleep-deprived to have a proper adult conversation or you end up talking about the baby all night long.
- First time you wear an ACTUAL bra that holds your boobs up, rather than a maternity bra (wait until breastfeeding is fully established).

AND WHEN IT ISN'T OKAY

Sometimes, despite it looking to the outside world like you're coping brilliantly, inside you might be feeling the complete opposite. And you need to take how you're feeling seriously. It is estimated that more than 1 in 10 women are affected with post-natal depression. Signs/symptoms may include:

- A persistent feeling of sadness and low mood.
- Lack of enjoyment and loss of interest in the wider world.
- Lack of energy and feeling tired all the time.
- Trouble sleeping at night and feeling sleepy during the day.
- Difficulty bonding with your baby.
- Withdrawing from contact with other people.
- Problems concentrating and making decisions.
- Frightening thoughts – for example, about hurting your baby.

If you're worried about how you're feeling, there are people to talk to and help is available. The most important thing to do is to speak to your midwife, health visitor or GP. Recognising that you may not be okay is the first step. Don't blame yourself, and don't think it will pass or maybe you're just tired.

I just kept crying and I didn't know why. I looked at my perfect baby and wonderful husband but I just felt so sad. I got really good at putting on an 'I'm fine' face and blamed my low mood on the broken nights. But as weeks passed, I isolated myself from friends and eventually my husband persuaded me to see my doctor. She was amazing. I just cried and she sat and listened. She didn't try and push anti-depressants on me but gave me treatment options. We need to be open about how we feel after having a baby; it's a life-changing event. We need to change society's stigma about mental health.

Rosie, mum of one

215

SO WHEN IS THE RIGHT TIME TO HAVE SEX?

The answer is: when you feel ready. That may be when your baby is 5 weeks old or when he or she is 5 months old. Only you know your body and how you feel, so don't feel pressured by others, or your partner for that matter. By the time you're thinking about having sex, you might have a vague idea of when your baby might be asleep for more than 10 minutes. Always pick a time when your baby has had a good feed, especially if you're breastfeeding (no one wants a leaky boob at a critical moment!) and has a clean nappy. There's nothing like having to change an up-the-back-leaked-all-over-the-clean-babygrow-type poo for killing the moment.

Your post-baby body isn't going to look how it used to. I remember being horrified when looking down at my stomach while in a certain position during sex with my husband after my first baby, thinking 'will it always hang down like that?' Obviously, with a bit of time and work it did eventually look marginally more acceptable, but it still wobbles and rolls in places.

> I think sex after birth is an oxymoron... It's terrifyingly wonderful. I was petrified of wiping myself after having a wee, let alone having a willy go there!! However, it's so lovely when you realise it all feels just as amazing and it helps to reunite you as a couple.
>
> *Lucy, mum of one*

Try not to ask your partner if it feels wider, bigger, looser, softer or different. It will put him off and kill the mood. You may feel different, but your partner may not even notice. He will just be pleased to be able to have some intimacy with you after such a long break.

The worst thing was the nerves. Would it hurt? What if I felt different or it wasn't enjoyable for either of us? It was like it was my first time all over again! It wasn't actually that bad or that uncomfortable; I think the fact that I was so tense was the biggest cause of discomfort. After lots of reassurance from my boyfriend and a few more goes I've got my confidence back, have relaxed and am enjoying it again.

Claire, mum of three

If you've had a C-section your vagina and perineum should feel and look the same as before you were pregnant, but you may still feel sore around your scar and your stomach muscles can still feel pretty wounded. A position like 'spoons' is probably sensible as it doesn't put any strain on your tummy. If you've had a vaginal birth obviously make sure your tear (if you had one) is completely healed before embarking on a passionate night in the bedroom. (At your six-week post-natal check-up with your GP, you can raise any issues you may have about your perineum and vagina.) You even may want to have a look with a mirror beforehand. Don't be freaked out by this idea. Getting to know what down there looks like is important for understanding how our bodies work and how well we heal after having babies. Go, Mother Nature! I have seen lots of women's vaginas after they've had an episiotomy or a second-degree tear and the tissues have healed really well.

- Only have sex when YOU feel ready.
- Choose a time when the baby is fed, clean and asleep.
- It's normal for the vagina to feel drier than usual after childbirth, which is linked to lower levels of oestrogen in your body compared to when you were pregnant. If you are breastfeeding they may be even lower: a water-based lubricant may help ease this.
- If it hurts or feels uncomfortable, just stop and try again another time.
- Choose positions that make you feel comfortable, so you can enjoy it.
- ALWAYS use contraception – even if you are breastfeeding (unless you want another baby straight away!).
- The more pelvic-floor exercises you do (see pages 58–9), the tighter your muscles will be (and the less likely you are to wet yourself on a trampoline!).

217

YOU'VE GOT THIS, MAMA!

Maternity leave can sometimes be boring, lonely and unfulfilling. And you may crave your old life and the job you left behind because you used your intelligent brain and felt stimulated and had proper lunch breaks and went for a wee without having a baby attached to you. But you are doing just fine. Who cares if your baby is wearing a stained babygrow and you haven't done the baby massage you were taught in those classes you paid for? All your baby knows and needs is you. And that can feel overwhelming too. You may feel like a failure and that you can't do it. You know in labour when you said 'I can't do this' and your partner and midwife said 'You can and you are doing this'? Well, remember that. Because all over the country and the world other mothers are thinking the same thing. You are scaling the mountain of motherhood. And no one said it was easy.

But the sleep does get better, and adjusting to motherhood takes time, plenty of time. Mine are nine, six and one and I'm still adjusting. Share your fears and anxieties with your mum-mates because we need to be sisterly in all of this – and be honest with one another.

And look, you've made it through the whole journey of pregnancy! I hope this book has helped you realise how amazing as women we are and what we go through to become mothers. It takes 40 (ish) weeks to grow a baby, so be kind to your body and don't expect it to snap back into shape. Remember that you grew a human and that is incredible!

But the journey doesn't end here, and it's wonderful and exciting and exhausting, but you're going to be just fine. You've got this, mama.